PRAISE FOR KATI MORTON

"A humane, compassionate, and extremely helpful guide to the complex world of mental health care. Knowing what's wrong and when to seek help can be life-changing, and Morton's book is packed with tools and tips for navigating life with mental health challenges."

—John Green, #1 *New York Times* bestselling author of *Turtles All the Way Down* and *The Fault in Our Stars*

"An exemplary guide for anyone wondering if they or someone close to them may benefit from mental health therapy."

—*Library Journal*

"An intuitive handbook that empowers readers to tend to their own mental health . . . Chapters provide practical tools for handling anxiety, depression, and other mental health difficulties, while also offering powerful insights."

—*Publishers Weekly*

"[Morton] answers the questions many of us have but don't necessarily feel comfortable asking. This is information everyone can benefit from."

—*Bustle*

"Compassionate and hopeful."

—*Energy Times*

"An undeniably essential read."

—*Cultured Vultures*

TRAUMATIZED

TRAUMATIZED

IDENTIFY, UNDERSTAND,
AND COPE WITH PTSD
AND EMOTIONAL STRESS

KATI MORTON, LMFT

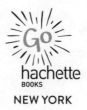

hachette
BOOKS

NEW YORK

Hachette Go, an imprint of Hachette Books
Hachette Book Group
1290 Avenue of the Americas
New York, NY 10104
HachetteGo.com
Facebook.com/HachetteGo
Instagram.com/HachetteGo

First Edition: September 2021

Hachette Books is a division of Hachette Book Group, Inc.

The Hachette Go and Hachette Books name and logos are trademarks of Hachette Book Group, Inc.

The publisher is not responsible for websites (or their content) that are not owned by the publisher.

Print book interior design by Trish Wilkinson.

Library of Congress Cataloging-in-Publication Data

Names: Morton, Kati, author.
Title: Traumatized: identify, understand, and cope with PTSD and
    emotional stress / Kati Morton, LMFT.
Description: First edition. | New York: Hachette Go, [2021] | Includes
    bibliographical references.
Identifiers: LCCN 2021008018 | ISBN 9780306924354 (hardcover) | ISBN
    9780306924347 (ebook)
Subjects: LCSH: Post-traumatic stress disorder. | Stress (Psychology) |
    Social media—Psychological aspects.
Classification: LCC RC552.P67 M684 2021 | DDC 616.85/21—dc23
LC record available at https://lccn.loc.gov/2021008018

ISBNs: 9780306924354 (hardcover), 9780306924347 (ebook)

Printed in the United States of America

LSC-C

Printing 1, 2021

To my patients and viewers who were brave enough to share their stories and teach me what it's really like to be traumatized. And to anyone who has ever felt like they were being too sensitive or alone with their pain. This book is for you.

CONTENTS

CONTENTS

AUTHOR'S NOTE

The people and patients I have discussed in this book have charitably given their permission. Many of the stories I share are very personal and come from those I know in my private life, as well as from my own life experience. To protect the privacy of those mentioned, all names and identifying details have been changed. The stories shared in this book are done to help further illustrate how mental health can affect us. This book is meant to empower you to get the help you need and deserve. It is not a replacement for actual mental health treatment. If you are struggling with mental health issues, I urge you to seek professional help as soon as possible.

INTRODUCTION

I have many goals for this book. Most important, I want it to help you more clearly understand what it means to be traumatized. I have been creating content online for over nine years and not a day goes by that someone doesn't message me asking if what they experienced is considered trauma or not. Most of us don't know the nuances and diagnostic criteria that help mental health professionals decide whether what someone is going through is a post-traumatic response. That information shouldn't be something we only have access to if we can afford to see someone. Trauma should be discussed openly, honestly, and done so often that if someone in our life goes through a terrifying situation, they feel empowered and supported enough to talk about and heal from it. My goal of getting mental health information out to those who need it has been the driving force behind my YouTube channel, my podcast, and now this book; if we don't have an understanding of trauma and how it's defined, how can we work to overcome it? We can't get help with something we don't know we have.

Having a name to put to what we feel can be validating and gives us a place to start when it comes to getting help. Information is empowering and gives us the language to frame our requests for support. This helps us figure out what type of mental health professional we are seeking and what to ask for when we make that first appointment. It can also help to know what the different trauma symptoms are, and how they can feel, so that we can more easily express what's going on to those who can help us. This can ensure we get useful tools and skills right away, and shorten the amount of time we spend in pain or feeling misunderstood. By walking you through all of this information, I hope you feel better prepared to ask for the help you need, want, and deserve.

I want you to know that I don't consider myself a trauma specialist. My career up until this point has focused on helping those with eating disorders and self-injury urges. I did most of my postgraduate work in an eating disorder treatment center and continued that work when opening my private practice. However, an interesting thing happened: As I helped my patients overcome their self-destructive urges, I began to realize that most of the reasons behind their desire to numb out or disappear grew out of their past trauma. Trauma was the common thread connecting these mental illnesses, and it was the root of the issues I was seeing each day. Without understanding it and how to treat it, I couldn't be an effective therapist, and I couldn't help my patients when they needed it most. It's because of this realization that I began to research trauma, and talk in depth about it with my online community, which inevitably drove me to write this book: so that anyone dealing with trauma or seeking more knowledge could find the answers and resources needed to help them on their path to recovery.

I hope that by offering therapeutic tools and techniques, as well as which styles of therapy are most effective, I am arming you with all you need to process what happened, begin healing, and be able to move past it to live the life you deserve. I also want the stories from my community to validate all you have been feeling and remind you that you are not alone in what you are going through. By shedding light on what trauma is and how it can feel, and by offering resources to help repair the damage, I hope more people feel seen, heard, and empowered to take their life back.

Surviving trauma is unimaginably difficult, and that can make it hard for us to see any good in the world. My goal is that this book is your much-needed reminder of the kindness still out there: that we can come together to validate one another's pain, connect through the heavy times, and share in healing knowledge and helpful resources. Today, we are more connected than ever before; let's use that to our advantage by sharing compassion, knowledge, and support.

TRAUMATIZED

CHAPTER 1

OUR SHARED TRAUMA

HOW SOCIAL MEDIA AFFECTS
OUR MENTAL HEALTH

T he past few years have been rough. We have encountered a world-
wide pandemic, witnessed multiple refugee crises, and America
has been at war for as long as most of us can remember. No matter what time of day we tune into news outlets, we are flooded with
frightening stories. We hear about various ecological disasters, sickness, riots, school shootings, and sexual assaults; the details and
images can be hard to take in and often impossible to forget.

This bombardment of information doesn't only happen through
traditional news outlets. Every day we see people sharing their
thoughts and experiences through YouTube, Facebook, Instagram,
Twitter, and more. Sometimes this content can be helpful and
exciting—connecting us with other cultures around the world and
allowing us to easily keep in contact with the people we love. However, there is a harmful side effect to all of this connection. Whether
it's videos of school shootings as they take place or interviews with
women speaking out about their experiences with sexual assault,
traumatic information is everywhere we look. It can feel impossible
to be online and not be inundated with terrifying information and
feel helpless to stop it.

Whether we realize it or not, this flood of negative information
takes its toll on our mental health. We can begin to see the world as a
scary and unsafe place, wonder whether we can trust our neighbors,

and possibly decide to not go out as much. Just the other day, I was walking to my local coffee shop when I heard a loud bang. I immediately considered my options: Should I run into this furniture store and hide there? Maybe I should dive into the alleyway? These thoughts were automatic, and all centered around my immediate belief that someone was shooting a gun in my neighborhood. I have never been to war or been anywhere near a terrorist attack, yet at that moment I believed I was in grave danger. This is the price we pay for being so connected and having access to upsetting images and information twenty-four hours a day, seven days a week.

Not to mention that because of COVID-19, we were told to stay home and stay safe; encouraged and often required to wear masks and stay at least six feet away from one another. I will personally admit that it did make me fear other people to some degree. I would worry about who has touched what, and whether I have sanitized things properly; I check and double-check my cleaning process because if I don't, I or someone I love could get sick, and without a treatment or vaccine available, it can feel like a matter of life and death. The constant stress of this pandemic, when all news outlets only cover the death tolls and the effect on our economy, has made it almost impossible to come out of this without some trauma response. In many ways I have felt like I can't look away, even if I try; the panic and upset are everywhere.

ARE THERE BENEFITS TO USING SOCIAL MEDIA?

I don't want you to think that social media is all bad, because there are many benefits to being connected. We can find other people who are just like us, reminding us that we are not alone, and that how we feel or what we think isn't weird or bad. Connecting can be freeing, validating, and it can improve our mental health. Many in my online community share how finding others with similar issues has been helpful, each sharing what has worked for them and supporting one another during the tough times. Instead of feeling like an outsider, we now have the tools to ensure we always find our peer group, even if they live on the other side of the world. It's powerful and life-changing.

We can also be inspired by other people in the world, seeing all that they are working on, the goals they set, and how they achieve it. This can help motivate those of us who are stepping out on our own without any road map or anyone nearby to help guide us. This connectivity can also encourage us to make a change outside of ourselves and in turn help others who may be going through a difficult time. We can help raise money for the fires in Australia or for a parent whose child is chronically ill by simply adding a Donate button to our posts. We can bring awareness to issues outside of our backyard by speaking up about it online, learning from one another as we share in experience and expertise. Being online can be helpful, supportive, and a medium for positive change, but we have to choose to use it that way.

The way we use social media is instrumental to our overall well-being. If we use it to connect and support, then we will feel those things in return. But if we use it to tear others down and spread hate and hurt, then we can start to think that that's all the world has to offer us. Being more mindful of what we do and who we follow online is key to ensuring social media has a positive effect on us. Everyone agrees that if you eat food devoid of any nutritional value, you won't feel as good as you would if you ate a nutritionally rich meal. The same goes for what you allow your eyes and mind to digest. Notice how you feel after reading or watching content online. Do you feel better or worse afterward? Are you jealous? Hate filled? Inspired or excited? Whatever you feel, pay attention to it. If you find yourself worse off emotionally after being online, it's time to reconsider what you are doing and who you are following.

I know all this talk about social media and mindfulness can seem silly or unimportant, but I assure you, it is neither of those things.

Just as with any new technological tool, we have to figure out how to use it in a way that is helpful, not hurtful; and part of this should be taking breaks from it altogether. I know you may have just audibly gasped or wondered why you picked up this book in the first place, but remember all things must be done in moderation. We have to listen to ourselves and make decisions that help us grow and change. If our social media practice is stressing us out, keeping us up, or feeding us negative thoughts about ourselves and our world, it needs to be adjusted.

HOW CAN WE IMPROVE OUR RELATIONSHIP WITH SOCIAL MEDIA?

The first step in adjusting our social media habits is to consider why we use it. Is it to unwind from a long day? Maybe it's to know what's going on with our friends and family? Or possibly we use it as a way to see what's happening in our world? Our reason could even change day-to-day or depending on how we feel. Take some time to think about why you use it, and then see whether that lines up with what you are getting out of it. If not, this may be a good time to plan a break from it or unfollow and mute accounts as needed. After a week or so of doing that, check back in with yourself to see whether things are more aligned and if you are feeling better.

If it's really difficult to put down your devices and take a real break, don't worry, you're not alone. In July 2019, the Pew Research Center polled American adults and found that more than 80 percent of them are online every day, with 28 percent of those polled stating that they are online "almost constantly."[1] I am even guilty of this. As someone whose business is primarily online, utilizing social media to reach more people, I would be hard-pressed to find a day when I wasn't online at least once, if not for most of the day. Trust me, I know what it's like and how hard it can be to not constantly check social media for fear that we will miss out on something. Newer research shows that the overuse of social media can lead to symptoms similar to substance-related addiction, some of which are marked changes in behavior, difficulty in relationships, and an inability to control use of social media.[2] Therefore, it may be increasingly difficult to break the habit of constantly checking our phone if we are in that 28 percent, but that doesn't mean we can't learn how to take breaks. Our breaks may look more like taking one night off every week or even just one hour away from our phones and other devices. The important thing is that we try to get off social media regularly so we can check in on ourselves and our mental health.

If we aren't able to change the way we interact with social media or at least work to manage the effects, we will continue to spread the trauma and upset we encounter while online. The sharing or spreading of trauma isn't a new concept; in fact, psychologists first noticed this in 1966, when most of their patients at the psychiatric clinic were children and grandchildren of Holocaust survivors.[3] They were shocked and couldn't figure out why such a large number of these people were seeking psychological support. They were dumbfounded because those seeking help didn't witness the trauma firsthand, they weren't the ones who were harmed during the Holocaust, so why did they seek out help? The truth is that these individuals had felt the effects of the Holocaust through their parents. It was passed down to them generation after generation, a phenomenon we call transgenerational trauma.

Even though I did not grow up in a Jewish home and I do not have any Holocaust survivors in my family, I do remember the effect the Great Depression had on my great-grandmother and my family. Whenever we would go out to dinner, she would stuff salt and pepper shakers as well as any leftover bread and butter into her purse before leaving. If I didn't want to take my leftovers home, she would have them boxed and shove those into her purse too. As a child I was embarrassed, and would always ask her what she was doing, sometimes pleading with her to stop. She never would, and instead would respond by saying, "Kati, they've got plenty here and you never know when you will need it, so it's best to save it now." My mom would try to explain to me why she did that and what she meant, but it wasn't until I was older and learned about the Great Depression that I understood her anxiety about not having enough to feed herself or her family.

Even if we take the word *trauma* out of this equation, think of how we pass down good behavior to our children. We demonstrate saying "please" and "thank you," and we instruct them to do it themselves when appropriate. Right? We teach using words and behaviors and repeat them until our children do it on their own. What happens if we refuse to let our children walk to the neighbor's house because "someone could hurt them" and jump every time we hear a loud noise? After a short while, our children can begin to feel unsafe walking on their own and startle every time they hear a car backfire.

That's not to say that we can't protect our children or show fear when scary things are happening; of course, we can do that! But what we need to be aware of is whether we are acting upon old unprocessed stories. I know that probably doesn't make sense, so let me explain what an old unprocessed story is. When we are traumatized or even really scared, our brain can't always make sense of the experience. It doesn't know how to put it into a full story and file it away into our memory. What happened can be too much for us to think about, process, and understand. So, these traumatizing memories never get dealt with; instead, they can remain scattered in our brain because we are never able to make sense of what occurred. All we know are bits and pieces of the event and what we learned from that.

This can lead to us believing certain things that simply aren't true. For example, let's say we were assaulted and robbed at gunpoint when we were twenty-two years old. What a terrifying thing to go through! How can we make sense of something that should never happen to a person? How can we even begin to process the fear we felt at that time? Without therapy, we may not be able to, and this can lead us to believe that it's never safe to walk down that specific street, or walk outside by ourselves, or possibly we could feel it's never safe to go outside again. Even though those responses can seem extreme, if we think about it, it does in some ways make sense. We were hurt on a particular street, by ourselves, and we were outside. If we don't take the time to piece together all that happened that day and understand that we can't always stop bad people from doing bad things, we can live our life from the perspective that if we just avoid the things we did that day, we won't be in danger ever again.

We can take this one step further and say that living through the lens of a traumatic memory would be akin to refusing to walk around anymore because one time we tripped and broke our leg. Sure, if we aren't walking around, it's not likely that we would trip or break our leg again, but we are also preventing ourselves from walking on the beach, traveling, or enjoying our life. We can even lead our children to believe that walking around in our world isn't safe and that they shouldn't do it either. The long-term effects of not understanding and processing our trauma aren't something we should take lightly. The confusion we may feel as the person experiencing the traumatic events, images, or videos is nothing in comparison to the upset our children could go through as a result.

One of the main reasons transgenerational trauma can be so hard to understand, let alone process through, is that the people it's passed down to didn't experience the trauma themselves. They don't have a story to process through with their therapist or a choppy memory to try to make sense of. All they have is a feeling, something they sensed from their caretakers that they can't put words to. It could have been the anxiety they felt when their mom gripped their hand tighter as they walked through town or the way their father's voice deepened as he spoke about certain times in his life. If the people we trust most express to us that something's wrong, we believe it without question or explanation.

Those of us with transgenerational trauma probably don't even know we have it. A lot of what we do as a result of this can seem normal or make logical sense to us. We learn so much from our parents and caretakers and often take their preferences or oddities at face value. I even buy certain brands of food at the grocery store because those are the ones that my grandma and mom always purchase. Have I tried the other brands, and decided these are superior? Nope. I just believe that they know best, and honestly, never questioned it. I only offer that example to demonstrate just how easily we follow what others in our family have done. We trust them, look up to them, and possibly want to be just like them. Not to mention that their way may be the only way we know, and if that's the case, how can we question something when we don't know of another option? We can't.

Trauma isn't just passed down; it can be passed across to our friends and others around us. This could be through images or stories we share online, or even through trying to help others. I frequently hear from first responders about how difficult and traumatizing their job is, and how they struggle to cope with it all. Even if we aren't the one who is hurt, seeing people who are hurting can be just as difficult to process. Do you ever watch the news or read an article about some horrific accident and have to look away or stop reading? Yeah, me too. It can be too much to handle sometimes and has even caused me to feel sick. That's because we are empathic people. We care about others and how they are doing. If someone is hurt or upset, we can feel somewhat responsible for what's going on and want to do everything we can to make it better.

That is yet another reason we need to be careful about what we see and say online. If we spend all day watching and reading content about people being unsafe, hurt, and horrible to one another, it's going to be hard for us to think about the world positively. I think we can all agree that the bad things are easier to believe and remember, but did you know that there's a reason for that? As adaptive creatures, we have to be constantly looking for any threat to our life. It's what keeps us safe and alive, and why our brain pays close attention to any warning or hazard. It wants to be sure that the scary thing isn't going to do us any harm. We observe and think through things until we are sure we can let them go. Which can feel like forever sometimes; trust me, I ruminate on negative things too.

Positive situations or thoughts, on the other hand, are not threatening, and for that reason, they are easy to ignore or forget. They can even be hard to pass down to our children or along to our friends because they aren't top of mind. That's why we need to constantly take stock of what we are allowing our brain to feast on, and sometimes force it to focus on the positive things.

The emotional ties we have to our families and friends can make this shared trauma difficult to stop. Sharing in experiences and beliefs is part of what connects us and gives us purpose and identity. If we don't feel connected to our family and friends, we can start to struggle with such thoughts as "Who am I?" "Where do I belong?" or "What do I believe?" Having others who think and act like us gives us a safe foundation from which we can grow and enter into relationships of our own. So, how do we keep the connection without spreading the trauma? It is a bit tricky, but with the right tools, we can handle it.

HOW DO WE STOP SPREADING THE TRAUMA?

In addition to identifying why we use social media and ensuring it lines up with what we get out of it, we also need to learn our limits—meaning that we can't live with rose-colored glasses on, or curate this idyllic environment and just forget what's going on in the world. Ignorance is bliss, but it can also lead to us being out of touch and putting ourselves in dangerous situations. Our goal shouldn't be to shut out anything upsetting or negative, but instead to work toward a more balanced view of the world. We can try to take in the good with the bad and manage how it's affecting us.

To strike this balance, we will need to first recognize our triggers. I know the word *trigger* has been overused and misunderstood in recent years, but triggers are real and can send us into a dark spiral if we aren't careful. That's why we must start to notice when something in our life triggers a trauma response. This could mean we find ourselves wanting to cry when we normally wouldn't or are extra jumpy when dealing with a certain person or situation. Being triggered means that something happening to us now has reminded us of something bad that happened before. This could be someone raising their voice to us at work, and it brings us back to when we were children and our mom would yell emotionally abusive things to us and our siblings. Or the smell of burning rubber reminding us of a terrible car accident we were involved in years ago.

Triggers can be any number of things depending on what we have been through, but they are usually connected to situations we haven't had the time to process through in therapy. It can involve any of our five senses and often feels like it comes out of nowhere. Since we can't control what we don't understand, I encourage you to think back to the last time you felt a little out of control or spaced out during a stressful time. Chances are, you were triggered in those moments, and the more you can recall about that day or week leading up to that feeling, the better you will be at identifying the thing or group of things that caused your trauma response.

Once we know what our triggers are, we can work to process through them as well as better manage our response in the moment. We can do these on our own, but it is easier and more productive if they're done with the help of a mental health professional—preferably, find one who specializes in trauma and understands how to best help us. They will help us figure out what is upsetting us, assist us in coming up with language to describe what happened, and talk us through the situation until it is no longer emotionally charged for us; that is, we will talk through the story or situation until it is no longer upsetting. Sure, it can still be described as sad or bad, but that doesn't change how we feel in the moment or ruin our entire day. This can take time, but it is honestly the best way to manage any past trauma and ensure we don't pass it on to our family or friends.

Next, we will have to find ways to take real breaks from being online. This doesn't mean we trade in our devices for our television, but that we aren't digesting any media from *anywhere*. As I mentioned earlier, I know this can be hard, and like any behavioral change, it will take time and practice. It may be best if we first plan to take some time off from our media when we are out to dinner or doing something else. That way we are distracted from the potential thoughts or urges that can come along with our first few social media breaks. It's completely normal to worry that we are missing out on things but, trust me, taking one night off isn't going to do any harm. There isn't any news feed, meme, or tweet that cannot wait a few hours. If something was an emergency that directly related to us, someone would call or text us.

I am going to be honest here: I am really bad at doing this. As I said, most of my work is online, and I struggle to not check my phone every few minutes; it's shameful really. But I was accidentally forced to quit cold turkey when I went camping with my family over the Memorial Day weekend. The cell service was so bad that I wasn't able to reload any of my social media apps or check my email. I couldn't do anything online for four whole days; it was my nightmare. But I had a choice to make: I could be upset, insist on going home, and ruin the trip for everyone, or I could suck it up and enjoy myself.

Of course, I sucked it up, but I was surprised at how quickly I forgot about my phone, social media posts, and keeping up with everything. I felt present, connected, and had a great time. Sure, I had the occasional thought to take a picture of this or that, but overall, I didn't even think about social media or what I was missing. I was busy doing my own thing, enjoying the lake, and relaxing with family, and I had the most recharging weekend of my adult life. Sadly, it took that experience to show me just how necessary these breaks are; just trust me when I tell you that it may be hard at first, but worth it.

Next, I want to talk about filtering our feeds. This is something that I do easily and often with reckless abandon, because it truly helps and is easy to do. But this shouldn't be done before we understand our triggers. Otherwise, we won't know which accounts to keep following and which ones to mute or unfollow. Here's how it works, once you have identified your triggers: If you find someone or some topic upsetting and difficult to stop thinking about, simply mute that person or type of content. As social media progresses, they continue to give us more tools to curate our feeds, so make sure you are utilizing these tools. I offer up the mute option because if the upsetting person is someone you know well, muting doesn't tell them you aren't following them anymore. You just don't see their feed, and you can always refollow or unmute things when you are feeling better, but you don't have to. Remember how I talked about paying attention to what we digest online? Make sure your feed is filled with things that are helpful and fulfilling for you.

Which rolls into my next tip, which is to check in with ourselves before and after using social media. If we are already feeling low or upset, now may not be the time to hop into our regular news feed; perhaps we could go for a walk or talk with a friend instead. It can be tempting to zone out and ignore what we are feeling but, trust me, that won't end up making us feel better. It can make us feel much worse. Just as our brain seeks out a threat and therefore can hold onto negative things, if we are already in a bad mind-set, we will most likely look for the hateful and hurtful things online because they validate how we already feel. Checking in with ourselves before engaging online allows us to decide whether we want to do it or not, whether we think it will be good for us. That way, we don't end up feeling worse and instead can make a more informed decision.

On the other hand, checking in with ourselves afterward can tell us how well we cleaned up our feed. When you are finished spending an hour or two online, how do you feel? Inspired? Informed and empowered? Or do you feel inferior, upset, and triggered? If you aren't getting what you need from your interactions online, you may want to go back to the previous step or take a break. Too often in life, we do things on autopilot without considering whether it's beneficial to us, and afterward, we are left wondering why we feel so bad. Taking a step back and considering what we are doing and how it's affecting us can change our mood and our outlook on life.

Since the news and other people's stories can cause us to feel helpless and hopeless, it's important to consider what we can and cannot control. I know this can be hard to do in the moment when something is upsetting and we feel the urge to help out or stop something from happening, but we don't always have that power. That's why it's helpful to take stock of what we *can* do, so we don't waste any time or energy fighting for things out of our control. Not to be the bearer of bad news, but in life, we can control only ourselves. I know we like to think that if we just do something a certain way or say the right thing, we can get people to do what we want. Wrong. Sure, we can get people to see things our way or persuade them to join us, but they are the ones that ultimately have control over their thoughts and behaviors. The sooner we let go of the illusion that we can make other people do things, the better.

When faced with something horrific and upsetting, consider what you can do. Can you donate money? Time? How about getting some like-minded people together to help petition for change? Setting up local meetings to share knowledge and raise money? There are so many things we can do to help out, and that's why we mustn't get caught up in trying to make other people do things too. Shouting at someone on Twitter isn't going to make them see things your way; only they can decide to change their mind, and in turn, change their behavior. Remember this tip when you find yourself saying things like, "I could get over this if only they would . . ." If we allow ourselves to think like that, we will be waiting on them forever. We can move past and process situations on our own, and no one has to change for that to happen.

We are bombarded daily with upsetting stories and images, and while most of these are correct and true, we must start checking the sources and facts. This isn't to say that everything posted on social media is made up, but it can often be skewed or biased in some way. At the risk of sounding completely stupid, I want to share a story about how I was fooled by a YouTube video last year, and how a simple fact-check could have saved me from myself. As I am sure you know, much of the news we get through our local outlets doesn't always cover world news, and therefore, I am often searching through YouTube to find out what else is happening in our world. After watching a video talking about a natural disaster happening in Southeast Asia, another video started playing. It looked like BBC News was reporting live about Russia invading Estonia. I was shocked, scared, and worried about the viewers I know who live in that area. I immediately put a clip on my social media, asking whether anyone knew anything about this and simultaneously did some research on it as well as checked to see who had posted the video. It turns out it was a fake, a joke of a video that someone created to show just how easily people would believe it.

I could have been angry at the person who had created the video, but I was mad at myself. I should have gotten my laptop out, looked up the title of the video, and checked to see who had created it. I should have done all of those things before sharing it online. I hate to think that my misstep could have upset or traumatized others, especially when a quick source check would have prevented it. I hope my mistake reminds you to check where your news is coming from before sharing or believing it to be true.

The last thing I want to talk about is that if you are trying some of the tips and you are still feeling overwhelmed, easily upset, or just as if you have unprocessed trauma, it is best to get into therapy. I know the idea of therapy can sound scary and we often think we have to be ill before talking to someone but, trust me, the sooner we get help, the better. We all have mental health that needs to be cared for, and our mental health is no different from our physical health. We wouldn't wait until we could barely get out of bed before we go see our doctor for a checkup, so why wait to see a therapist? A therapist can help you figure out what is causing your trauma symptoms and give you therapeutic tools to better manage them. Just make sure you find one you connect with, who makes you feel heard and understood.

Technology has changed how we interact with our world, but that doesn't mean we can't find ways to ensure this new way of communicating is healthy and helpful. Instead of mindlessly scrolling, taking in information, and not considering the effects it can have, I hope we can all be more mindful and engage with purpose. As with any change we try to make in life, it will take time and practice, and there will still be days where we want to dive into a news article even though we know it could upset us. If you are still wondering whether your social media use is healthy or unhealthy, here is a quick questionnaire:

- Do you spend more than five hours a day online? Or check your phone constantly?
- Do you find yourself getting into heated arguments online? Or wanting to leave hate-filled comments or responses?
- After being online, do you feel worse? Or more negative about life and the world around you?

- Do you have a hard time taking a break from checking or interacting on social media?
- Do you find yourself being jealous or upset by those you follow, but struggle to unfollow them?

If you answered yes to more than one of those questions, it may be beneficial to reassess your social media use, take another look at the tips I offered, and make some changes. Social media should be something we use to connect with others, learn from differing perspectives, and be reminded that we are not alone. Making some changes to how we use social media can benefit not only our mental health, but those around us too. I hope that if we are all more aware, and doing our best to use social media for good, we can stop the gratuitous spread of trauma and instead work to heal ourselves.

CHAPTER 2

HAVE I BEEN TRAUMATIZED?

PTSD & WHAT YOU NEED TO KNOW

W hen we hear the words *post-traumatic stress disorder* (PTSD), it's common to automatically think of our veterans and those who have been affected by war in one way or another. PTSD used to be known as "shell shock," and later as "combat stress reaction," both of which were terms used by the Veterans Administration to describe the symptoms experienced by over eighty thousand World War I soldiers.[1] Since the diagnostic criteria for PTSD didn't exist yet, soldiers came up with these terms to describe why they or their fellow troops couldn't function in their combat roles anymore even though they were physically able. Many struggled to sleep due to intense nightmares. Others would freeze in combat, putting themselves and those around them in danger. These symptoms were affecting so many troops that it was hindering the British Army's ability to fight in the war, and so they hired psychologist Charles S. Myers to study the issue in hopes of finding a way to treat or manage it.[2]

Myers began to study soldiers who reported having shell shock and found that they seemed to view themselves and their situation very differently from those around them. Many were fatigued, struggled to keep their balance, had tremors, and reported headaches. Alongside another psychologist, William McDougal, Myers hypothesized that these symptoms were arising due to the suppression of the trauma of war. They believed that by talking about the trauma and helping it be integrated into the patient's conscious mind, the shell shock symptoms would subside.[3] Although the war was terrible and traumatizing to many, it was the beginning of trauma research and why we have the information and understanding that we do today.

While Myers and McDougal believed they had a treatment option for those suffering soldiers, the real struggle was in testing it and making it quick enough to be integrated into the army bases. After testing these new methods on a few soldiers, they found that their hypothesis was correct, and integrative therapy techniques did alleviate the shell shock symptoms. The next hurdle was the volume of need and trying to find a way to apply these therapeutic techniques at scale. The closer they were to the action, the faster they could get the soldiers into treatment and back out in the field, and so they urged the armed forces to create special units close to their bases where they could quickly treat any troops experiencing the symptoms of shell shock. They believed that with swift therapeutic interventions, they could prevent the symptoms from getting worse, and get the soldiers back to their posts quickly. The armed forces must have thought his methodology was successful as they still use this treatment plan in war zones today.[4]

While those who have been in combat still suffer from the symptoms of PTSD, it's not something that only soldiers can struggle with. In Dr. Bessel van der Kolk's wonderful book *The Body Keeps the Score*, the author explains that one does not have to be a combat soldier, or visit a refugee camp in Syria or the Congo, to encounter trauma. He cites research by the Centers for Disease Control and Prevention showing that one in five Americans is sexually molested as a child; one in four is beaten by a parent to the point of a mark being left on their body; and one in three couples engages in physical violence. A quarter of us grew up with alcoholic relatives, and one out of eight witnessed their mother being beaten or hit.[5]

While those statistics may sound shocking or impossible, believe me when I tell you that they are real. I hear about it every day and work tirelessly alongside those who have been traumatized as they make their way toward healing. I know it's hard to take in and understand, as it's human nature to not want to hear about trauma or upset. Listening to how someone was harmed as a child can be difficult, and imagining a person who would do such harm can threaten our belief in our fellow man. Unfortunately, trauma is all around us, happening each day, and that's why we must understand what it is and how it can feel.

HOW IS PTSD DIAGNOSED?

The first thing to know about PTSD is that we can suffer from the symptoms even if the event didn't happen directly to us. The *Diagnostic and Statistical Manual of Mental Disorders*, 5th edition (*DSM*-5), states:

> Exposure to actual or threatened death, serious injury, or sexual violence in one (or more) of the following ways:
>
> 1. Directly experiencing the traumatic event(s).
>
> 2. Witnessing, in person, the event(s) as it occurred to others.
>
> 3. Learning that the traumatic event(s) occurred to a close family member or close friend. In cases of actual or threatened death of a family member or friend, the event(s) must have been violent or accidental.
>
> 4. Experiencing repeated or extreme exposure to aversive details of the traumatic event(s) (e.g., first responders collecting human remains; police officers repeatedly exposed to details of child abuse).[6]

Therefore, even if a threatening event happens to someone we are close to, we, too, can be affected by it. The *DSM* does add a caveat to the fourth criterion, stating that it "does not apply to exposure through electronic media, television, movies, or pictures unless this exposure is work-related." While I understand where the manual's writers were coming from when they added that caveat, I have to adamantly disagree. When this new edition of the *DSM* came out in 2013, social media, livestreaming, and even the news wasn't what it is today. Not to mention that the people who work on such literature are most likely not engaging in social media, and may not understand its development and reach. Instead, they focus their attention on analyzed research papers and other published articles on the subject. In short, our research will never catch up with the ever-changing media landscape, and will always fall short of integrating it into the diagnosis and treatment of mental illnesses. Which is why things like the *DSM* and other manuals are helpful when learning about diagnoses, their prevalence, and comorbidities, but are not the only information one needs to consider. I believe that the best tool we have for understanding and treating mental illnesses is our patients and their stories, and by listening to them and letting them lead us through their experience, then and only then can we give them proper treatment.

Since I do believe that diagnostic criteria are important to the basic understanding of a diagnosis, let's dig into the actual diagnosis of PTSD. Once we or someone we love has seen or experienced a traumatizing event, it must be followed by intrusive memories of the event, avoidance of anything that reminds them of the event, a more negative outlook on their life and the world around them, and changes to how they react and respond to life. A diagnosis of PTSD can also be accompanied by dissociative symptoms, but not in all cases.[7]

I know that's a lot of information and symptoms to understand, so let's break it down a bit. First, we have the intrusive symptoms, which are most commonly called flashbacks. These can happen when we are awake and triggered by something in our environment, such as a smell or sound. A flashback isn't always just a quick clip of a traumatizing time flashing in our mind; it can cause us to feel as if we are back in the place where the event occurred and that the trauma is happening to us or our loved one again. In many ways, I feel that flashbacks continue the trauma experience and can perpetuate our symptoms of PTSD almost as if we are caught in a loop of trauma experience of cope or repress, and experience the trauma again. These flashbacks can also happen while we sleep, taking the form of a nightmare, again causing us to feel that we are back in that terrorizing situation. Many of my patients and viewers have shared how the nightmares make it impossible for them to sleep, and they wake up screaming or covered in sweat. Since trauma memories are not always clear or linear, flashbacks can also feel like flipping through a photo album where certain situations are frozen in a still frame, and as we move through the flashback, it flips from one photo to another.

Avoidance is the set of PTSD symptoms that logically make the most sense. We avoid things that we don't want to deal with, and if we expect to continue our life post-trauma, then we are going to have to avoid all things that trigger us. For a second, imagine that you were physically and emotionally abused as a child, and therefore anyone raising their voice can send you into a flashback. This can make it impossible for you to focus and do your job, not to mention that you may have to go outside or home to calm yourself down. Now, let's say that you just started a new job, and as we learn about protocols and procedures, you make a mistake, and your boss yells at you. For some people, this would be upsetting, but they'd probably just feel bad and promise to do better next time. But if you have a history of trauma relating to yelling and loud voices, this could be so debilitating that it could cause you to quit your new job immediately. You would want to avoid that type of situation or behavior because it's simply too distressing for you to manage.

My biggest issue with avoidance is when we not only avoid certain situations or people, but we take it to the next level by avoiding specific thoughts, memories, feelings, or anything that we think is linked to our trauma. We stuff it down deep into ourselves and try to forget that it's there at all. This makes sense when we are in a hurtful situation, as it allows us to keep going, push through, and survive it. However, when we are free from those circumstances, keeping it in will only make us feel worse. Which leads us into the final two sections of symptoms.

First up is memory loss related to the traumatic situation—meaning that we can't recall much about a certain time in our lives or a specific experience. I have heard from patients, viewers, and even close friends that they have no memory of years of their upbringing because it was so tumultuous. Many worry that maybe they are making it all up because they only remember a few small bits of a situation, or that it wasn't that bad because what they remember was just moderately upsetting. Memory loss due to stress or trauma, called dissociative amnesia, is the biggest struggle when we are trying to heal. I mean, think about it: How can we heal from something we can't remember? How do we know we aren't making up the memories as they slowly come back? This is one of the most substantial reasons that I recommend working with a mental health professional, and if available, one who specializes in trauma. They can offer tips and tools and ways to encourage our memory to come back while having us fact-check things along the way.

Along with memory loss, stuffing down our feelings can also lead us to think of people and our world as a negative and unsafe place. We can struggle to connect with others, not want to engage in social activities, and feel unable to have any positive thoughts. It's also common to turn those negative thoughts on ourselves, believing that the trauma was our fault and we did something to cause it. These thought spirals can lead us to believe that we will never be able to get better and are ruined for life. We don't want to see real pain or hear about how common child abuse is; we would prefer to think of our communities and our country as a safe and kind place. So, it's no wonder we struggle to cope with trauma, wanting to shove it deep down and pretend it didn't happen, but when it pops back up to remind us it's there, begging to be dealt with, we can think that something is wrong with us. We can believe that if we were stronger, we wouldn't have to process it; that we could just move on. We need to know that there isn't anything wrong with us: Our trauma just needs to be seen and heard from so that it can be processed and filed away with our other memories. Stuffing things down only hurts us and hinders our future; whereas, by acknowledging our pain and trauma, we can let it go.

Possibly the most noticeable set of symptoms are those of over-reaction. These can include hypervigilance, irritability, struggling to concentrate, engaging in reckless or self-destructive behavior, and being easily startled.[8] I have always hated the term *overreaction* because I think it's been given a bad rap over the years, often connected with someone being unstable or irrational, but I don't see it that way. Overreaction is something we do because we don't see another way of responding. We may not know how to take a beat, breathe, and then figure out what to do. This doesn't mean we aren't capable of learning how to respond versus react, and as a therapist, I am always very curious and interested in an overreaction. It tells us something else is going on that is taking away our ability to see things clearly, and trauma is one of the things that can cause an overreaction.

The last potential criterion for PTSD is dissociation. In response to the trauma, we can experience depersonalization and/or dereal-ization, which are forms of dissociation. Either form can occur when our brain simply cannot stay present and process what's happening, so it allows us to float away for a bit to catch up with all we may be experiencing. Depersonalization is when we feel detached from ourselves. Many of my viewers and patients say it's like being a ghost of ourselves, almost as if we're floating above our body, watching it go through all of our daily tasks and motions. Then there's dere-alization, where we feel detached from our surroundings, or as if we are in a dream. This has been described to me as more distant or severe than depersonalization because we are not just outside of ourself but outside of our environment, and what's around us can even be distorted in color or shape. Since I haven't experienced either of these, I can't say which is worse or better, just that they are a sign from our brain that what we are going through is too much for it to process. It needs a break from reality so it can get caught back up.

BEYOND THE DIAGNOSTIC CRITERIA
FOR TRAUMA—BIG Ts AND LITTLE Ts

I don't want you to think that the diagnostic criteria are all that I consider when diagnosing someone with PTSD. As I shared before, it's my patient's stories and experiences, as well as my own, that help guide us in our journey to healing. One thing I have learned through my time online and in practice is that not all traumas start out as traumatic. What I mean by that is, on its own, a certain experience could not be seen or felt as a trauma. Perhaps it was simply an upsetting event that we were able to think about, feel out, and be done with. However, when we start stacking these smaller yet troubling events on top of one another, possibly back-to-back, without giving us the time to think about them and process how we feel, they can grow into a trauma.

We call these smaller upsetting situations "little Ts," and the other, more immediately traumatizing situations "big Ts." This has been helpful in my practice when trying to better understand my patient's symptoms and experiences. Too often I hear how there hasn't been anything big that happened, such as abuse or a car crash, and therefore there is no reason for their PTSD symptoms. Not knowing why we feel the way we feel can not only be painful and invalidating, but can also cause us to believe that there's something bigger wrong with us. To further explain what big Ts and little Ts are, I reached out to my friend and colleague Dr. Alexa Altman, who is, in fact, a trauma specialist and the person who introduced me to these terms.

A big-T trauma is distinguished as an extraordinary and potentially life-threatening event that leaves a person feeling powerless and out of control. Some examples of big-T traumas are severe car accidents, near drowning, exposure to war, natural disasters, physical assault, etc. After a big-T trauma, a person will often report feeling terror, rage, a fear of death, helplessness, a loss of faith in god, or a loss of faith in humanity. A big-T trauma can be analogized to a tsunami. When a tsunami wave pummels the shore, it engulfs everything in its path, swallowing it whole and pulling it back out to sea. Like a tsunami, a big-T trauma can obliterate a person's psychological and physical constitution destroying a sense of self, personal identity, and purpose.

Whereas, little-T traumas are events that surpass a person's capacity to cope and can disrupt emotional, social, and cognitive functioning. These events may not be life-threatening but are extremely stressful and pose a threat to one's sense of emotional well-being. Some examples of small-T traumas are employment loss, divorce, chronic illness, interpersonal conflict, and legal challenges. Calling a very challenging event "little" can be dismissive or discount the negative impact of these stressful life events. A little-T trauma can be analogous to a large wave at the beach. When confronted by one big wave, holding the breath, ducking under a wave, one can still regain footing on the other calmer side of the swell. But, what happens when these waves come in rapid succession? The ability to catch one's breath and regain a solid stance is diminished. The next stressful event or wave will be experienced much harder than if a full recovery was possible. The cumulative effect of small-T traumas can be overlooked by an individual or even a clinician. Thus the accumulation of small-T events can actually lead to a big T, leaving a person unable to comprehend why a common stressful event can feel so crippling.

Just this year, I had a close friend reach out to share how she was struggling with dissociation and hypervigilance for the past two years but couldn't figure out why. She had a pretty normal and happy childhood; both of her parents were still in her life and they all got along; she had had a few long-term relationships throughout the years, but again, no abuse or trauma there. I remember her lamenting to me after a long phone call about how she wished she had just been in a car accident or something so it would all make sense. I felt helpless to shed some light on what she was experiencing until I learned about little Ts a few months later. So, I called her and asked whether there had been any smaller yet still upsetting situations in the past two or three years. After racking our brains, we came up with a whole slew of smaller Ts: She had received a promotion at work three years ago and was relocated; while it was exciting, it was also upsetting because she had to move farther from her friends and family. The following summer, her grandmother passed away, and not two months later, so did her grandmother on the other side of the family. A few months after all of that, one of her long-term relationships abruptly ended, and that's when the symptoms began. There we had it, a timeline filled with little Ts all building up until she couldn't process anymore, and that's when the dissociation and hypervigilance began.

While that wasn't one of the happiest phone calls I have had, it was exciting because we were able to unearth the reason behind it all and in a way explain her symptoms. Of course, I recommended that she see a trauma therapist as soon as possible, and she is still working on those little Ts, but I am happy to report that her dissociation barely happens anymore! This is a nice reminder that with proper support and treatment life can get better.

I am sure even the thought of little Ts has you searching your memory for any inkling of trauma or upset, so here is a quick questionnaire to help you decide whether you have been through a trauma or not.

- Have you had various stressful events occur within the last six months or up to a year?
- Have you struggled to function in your daily life? Maybe unable to be social or go about your day without getting emotional?
- Have you recently been through some major life change? Such as moving, going through a divorce, or getting married?
- Have you had changes to your job situation? Like losing or getting a new job? Or perhaps you have retired recently? Are you struggling financially?
- Are you struggling with any ongoing interpersonal conflict? Fights with a spouse or family member? Ending of a long-term friendship?
- Do you or someone you love live with a chronic illness? Or have you lost a loved one recently?

If you said yes to more than one of these questions, it's possible that you have been exposed to some little-T traumas, and seeing a mental health professional to work through it could be beneficial. The sooner we get support for all we go through in life, the better we will feel and the more easily we will be able to manage the next upset.

KEY TAKEAWAYS

- Post-traumatic stress disorder (PTSD) isn't something that affects only soldiers or veterans.

- PTSD can be diagnosed if we or someone we love has been in a terrorizing and traumatizing situation. We can have flashbacks about this experience, avoid anything that reminds us of it, and be constantly on guard to prevent it from happening again.

- Memory loss is very common when we have been through a traumatic experience.

- We can have dissociative symptoms on their own or as part of our PTSD.

- Make sure your mental health professional rules out other diagnoses before settling on a PTSD diagnosis.

- Mental health professionals should let their patients be the real resource when putting together a plan for treatment.

CHAPTER 3

WHAT CAN CAUSE PTSD?

There are many various causes for PTSD and no way to list them all, which is why I prefer instead to focus on the way we talk about PTSD and define what trauma is. The most inclusive and understanding definition I can come up with is that trauma is anything that happens to you or someone else that is too much for your brain to process at the moment. The sheer exposure to the situation pulls you out of a calm or relaxed state and pushes you into either fight, flight, or freeze mode (otherwise known as your stress response). I like to think of PTSD in that way because it takes into consideration what each person can handle, validating everyone's experience and potential resulting symptoms.

That definition is also important when dealing with group trauma. It can help someone understand why they were so traumatized by a situation when their older sibling wasn't. I hear about things like this all the time, how two siblings went through the same situation, yet one is fine and the other is grappling with symptoms of PTSD. This discrepancy could have to do with their age, emotional maturity, or ability to cope on their own, and we are seeing this play out right now in the wake of COVID-19. Some people are taking the pandemic in stride, deep cleaning their house, making sourdough bread, and planting a garden, whereas others are struggling to get out of bed, shower, or take care of their basic needs. Everyone's ability to cope is different, and there shouldn't be judgment surrounding that. We wouldn't judge someone for catching a cold when the rest of us happened to not get it, so why would we treat mental illness any differently?

If you are not sure whether PTSD is what you or someone you love is experiencing, it's best to see a mental health professional so they can properly assess what's going on and ensure you get the right treatment. Also, if you are still wondering whether you need to see a trauma specialist, here is a quick questionnaire that should help:

- Do you think you have been exposed to a traumatic experience?
- Do you often feel that your emotions are out of control?
- Do you frequently have flashbacks or bad dreams related to the traumatic event?
- Do you view others or the world around you as bad or unsafe?
- Do you find yourself numbing out from all you are feeling with drugs, alcohol, gambling, or shopping?

If you answered yes to two or more of these questions, it's worth finding a mental health professional who specializes in trauma. That will ensure that instead of being pulled off course by other symptoms, they will view all of your symptoms as part of the bigger issue, the trauma, and possible PTSD. In my years of experience, I cannot emphasize enough how important it is that we get to the root of our issues in therapy. I know that sounds obvious, but what I mean by that is we can't get distracted by every new symptom, spending our time trying to keep them all at bay. That would be like going to the doctor because of a stomach upset, and instead of running a test to see what's causing it, they treat only our nausea and send us on our way. After a day or two, we would find ourselves back in their office still not feeling well. Sure we need to deal with those symptoms, but if we can figure out what's causing the pain and digestion issues and heal that, the other problems will subside too. In therapy, we want to manage the symptoms that are bothering us, but to stop them from continuing to come back day after day, we need to focus on the root cause and process that through. Otherwise, we've only treated the surface issues, and the real problem has yet to be identified and dealt with.

ARE YOU SURE IT'S PTSD?

When working on a diagnosis with a patient, mental health professionals are trained to complete what is called differential diagnosis, which is when we rule out other possible diagnoses to ensure that PTSD is in fact what we are dealing with. While I walk you through all of the signs and symptoms of PTSD, I am sure you will see that depending on how it presents, it could look like a lot of other mental illnesses. For example, if someone has a negative outlook on life and reports issues with their sleep, it could be major depressive disorder (MDD). To distinguish between these two diagnoses, we would have to check to see whether they have any flashbacks, dissociation, or hypervigilance, and if they do, then it's most likely PTSD, not MDD.[1]

Another group of disorders that could look and feel a lot like PTSD are adjustment disorders. These require a stressor, just like PTSD; however, when it comes to adjustment disorders, the stressor can be any intensity; it doesn't have to be threatening or traumatizing. If we were upset by our spouse leaving us, and going through the divorce proceedings causes us to become irate in public, and we avoid all things that remind us of them, we could think we are struggling with PTSD. However, we are missing a lot of the symptoms of PTSD, such as hypervigilance, flashbacks, and a negative outlook on the world. Moreover, if our symptoms go away after six months or so, it's most likely an adjustment disorder.

You see, adjustment disorders occur when we are going through a period of difficulty and change, such as a divorce, a move, change of job or school, or anything that adds to the stress of our life. We can struggle to function, and if we were able to look at the situation objectively, we would agree that our reaction to the situation is out of proportion with what's going on. Once we feel more settled and adjusted, these symptoms go away. If we have been exposed to something traumatizing, and do have such symptoms as flashbacks or struggle to remember the details, it's more likely that what we are experiencing is PTSD.

Acute stress disorder is yet another diagnosis that shares some of the same symptoms of PTSD and should be ruled out before moving forward with treatment. The difference between these two diagnoses is pretty simple: with acute stress disorder, the symptoms last anywhere from three days to one month following the traumatic event.[2] Any longer than that indicates that it can't be acute stress disorder and must be something else, such as PTSD.

Because a potential symptom of PTSD is dissociation, it's also important to rule out dissociative disorders. The real way to ensure that what's going on is PTSD and not a dissociative disorder is to see whether the individual has all or most of the symptoms of PTSD, not just dissociation. Those who struggle with dissociation do not always have PTSD, so we need to check whether they have flashbacks, exposure to a terrifying or traumatizing event, and many other parts of the PTSD diagnosis. If not, and their main symptom is dissociation, then we would want to explore those to see which dissociative disorder fits best.

For a while, I thought that the COVID-19 pandemic was going to throw most of us into acute stress disorder, PTSD, or possibly an adjustment disorder. We were faced with a terrifying virus and illness that we don't know how to treat, not to mention that we have to adjust to being at home more and not out in public places with friends and family. The transition has been difficult and upsetting, causing people to struggle with increased anxiety, have depressive thoughts, and even to develop a negative outlook on their life and world. There have been numerous incidents of people getting into physical altercations with police and security guards because of the new laws and regulations around where they can go and what they can do. It's been incredibly hard.

However, as things continue to unfold, I have realized that each person will react differently. Some may experience PTSD if they or someone they care about was harmed by COVID-19 or any of the side effects it's caused. Others may struggle to adjust to the "new normal" and be upset for a few months, whereas some may have some PTSD symptoms but those last for only a few weeks. Again, everyone's ability to cope is going to be different, but everyone's affected.

I recently read a post by someone I have been following online for years. She was sharing how her husband had caught the coronavirus and due to many complications, he had to be put into a medically induced coma. She was devastated: they had just had a new baby, he was only forty-one, and he was healthy with no preexisting medical conditions. How could this happen to him? To her? I sat staring at my phone in tears, hurting for them and their family, for the loss and trauma they were experiencing. I even had dreams about it, waking up in the middle of the night upset as if it were happening to me. Sure, you could say that I am just being sensitive and that I don't know this person outside the online community, but trust me when I tell you that I was deeply upset by her story and situation. In part, I think this is because I, too, am affected by the virus; it's changed my life and my outlook on the world. In a way, I think I can imagine what she must be going through because I am going through a minuscule version of it, and I am connected to her online. So again, when I read in the *DSM* that you cannot have PTSD through electronic media, I have to disagree. We are linked, we feel that we know one another, and in many ways, we can share in the trauma. I also offer this example in hopes that it validates anything you have been feeling during the pandemic. Too often we assume that how we think and feel is unique or odd; however, it's all normal and okay as long as we do our best to offer compassion and understanding to one another as we navigate this new world.

Finally, I want to address the small difference between how adults versus children experience PTSD. In children six years old and younger, along with experiencing the trauma themselves, they can also be traumatized by seeing or hearing of their parent or caregiver being hurt. Since we rely so much on those who care for us when we are young, it is devastating to have anything happen to them. Although the *DSM* doesn't have this criterion, I want to add that in my professional experience, children tend to developmentally regress when traumatized. This could cause them to start sucking their thumb again, not be able to sleep alone, or even wet the bed after being potty trained. I have always believed that this was because they were trying to go back to a time when they felt safe and okay, or possibly because they feel that growing up only means more danger is there, so they would rather not. Whatever the reason, I personally always ask questions about this to ensure I am not missing one of these important red flags.

WHY DIAGNOSIS ISN'T EVERYTHING

When I was getting my master's degree back in 2008 I used to pore over the *DSM* as if it was the Bible. I would read about different diagnoses, their corresponding symptoms, and what I needed to rule out before making a diagnosis. Even in my work on YouTube, I utilize the *DSM* for most videos, citing it, reading from it, and helping it guide how I talk about certain mental illnesses. Although it does help give some guidance and a place to start when considering someone's symptoms, it can also box me in and cause me to overlook certain issues because it doesn't fit with what the *DSM* says.

The first time I realized that the *DSM* could be limiting was when I was working with my first eating disorder patient. She had a slew of symptoms, everything from panic attacks, depressive thoughts, and purging behaviors to even some nonsuicidal self-injury. She came to me asking for help with her eating disorder issues, but so many other things were going on and I was at a loss as to where to start. So, I asked my supervisor for some help, pulling out my handy-dandy *DSM* in the process and opening it up to the section about borderline personality disorder (BPD). He pushed my book shut, telling me not to rely so heavily on it, and to instead look at my patient: What were her biggest complaints? What symptoms was I the most worried about? Did I have any idea where all of these symptoms could be coming from? He encouraged me to start there, ask her more questions, and let her teach me about her experience, instead of trying to squeeze her issues into a diagnostic box. It was eye-opening, and I am still thankful for his insight so early on in my career. It helped me treat my patient as the unique person she was and cater to her needs, instead of trying to rush to diagnose.

I would like to say that I learned my lesson after that one conversation, but it was programmed into me to use that manual as a guide for treatment, and so I found myself struggling with a similar situation about a year later. I was working with a young man who came in for help with his anxiety. He was successful in business, had done well in school, and even had a thriving social life. On paper, his life looked great and without issue. After working with me for a while, he confided that he had, on occasion, self-injured. If I am being honest, I was surprised. He had everything working for him and we had finally gotten his panic attacks under control. Why was he self-injuring? The only diagnosis at the time that included self-injury was borderline personality disorder, but he didn't have any of the other symptoms. I remember digging through my trusty *DSM* after that session, trying to make sense of this remaining symptom, looking for something I missed. Then, I remembered what my first supervisor said, don't get caught up in the criteria, let your patient teach you. And so I asked more questions, sought to understand his experience, and learned that the self-injury was one of the ways he dealt with all of his anxiety, and even though some of the tools we had worked on were helpful, nothing helped as much as that. So, after a particularly stressful day, he would still struggle to fight the urges to harm himself. If I hadn't taken the time to ask about it, I could have not only misdiagnosed him but also started down a path of treatment that didn't fit his issues.

You see, the *DSM* never taught me that self-injury could be a coping skill and doesn't always have to be part of a BPD diagnosis. Instead, the *DSM* labels each issue, pushing everyone into boxes, organizing each symptom as part of a flow chart leading you to what it believes the diagnosis should be. As much as I enjoy organization and flow charts, this was only making my professional life harder, and while I still reference it when needed, I have decided that my patients are the best manual, and I should lean into them as much as possible.

Another issue I have with the *DSM* is how it seems to refuse to include how situations and relationships can impact people. When reading through the PTSD diagnosis, you will see a small portion entitled "Risk and Prognostic Factors" that includes pre-traumatic factors, peritraumatic factors, and post-traumatic factors. All in all this information doesn't even take up half a page. In that short space, it covers genetic predispositions, environmental factors, and how someone's temperament can affect their mental health. I don't know about you, but I feel that instead of spending all our time talking about symptoms, we should be focused on the causes, because it's in those that we can find the cure. For starters, the environmental factors should be woven throughout the diagnostic criteria since it's something in our environment that traumatizes us, and having social support (another environmental factor) is paramount to our development and recovery.

Going back to what I said about treating the root of the issue instead of just the symptoms, I believe we focus too much on the symptoms and not enough on the environment that's causing them. If we all take a minute to think about any mental health issue we've ever had—feeling anxious, being overly stressed, or having depressive thoughts—we can always pinpoint at least one thing in our environment that either caused or exacerbated it. I hope that we move our schooling and continuing education away from the *DSM* and symptoms and into a more holistic view, because nothing in our life happens in a vacuum. All health professionals should be taught to consider relational and environmental factors while tracking the reported symptoms; in doing so, I believe we could all find more understanding and healing instead of just diagnoses.

While I am not interested in getting involved in the politics of diagnosis, and what we should or shouldn't use, I do think it's important to know that the *DSM* and any other manual cannot possibly address all human experience. Therefore, if you read through the symptoms we discussed and felt that many issues were left out or part of your experience wasn't mentioned, that's a failing on our system, not on you. Our system should support referencing criteria while focusing the majority of our time and energy on listening and learning from our patients. Our patients should be our road map to treatment and healing.

KEY TAKEAWAYS

- Trauma can be defined as anything that happens to us or someone else that is too much for our brain to process at the moment.

- In addition to being exposed to a traumatizing event, the likelihood of us being traumatized is linked to our level of resistance, and can be affected by our age, emotional maturity, or capacity to cope on our own.

- PTSD can look a lot like major depressive disorder (MDD), various adjustment disorders, acute stress disorder, and some dissociative disorders. That's why it's vital that we are properly assessed by a mental health professional.

- Children six years old and younger can be traumatized by seeing or hearing of their parent or caregiver being hurt, because they rely on them for much of their care and support.

- Not all experiences and struggles will fit within the diagnostic criteria, but that doesn't mean we don't deserve help.

CHAPTER 4

WHAT IS DISSOCIATION & WHY DOES IT HAPPEN?

E xperiencing a traumatic event can lead to dissociative amnesia, which is when we cannot remember the details or possibly any portion of what happened to us. This can be distressing and has led many of my patients to believe that they are making up their symptoms of PTSD, but dissociative amnesia isn't the only form of dissociation out there. We can feel spaced out, daydream, and even completely disconnect from our body, and it's believed that roughly half of all adults have experienced at least one of these episodes.[1] They are part of what's called dissociative disorders and the *DSM* places them next to the trauma and stress-related disorders to reflect how closely connected, although separate, they are from one another.

When something overwhelming or traumatic occurs in our life, it can be too much for our brain to sort through or make sense of. It can be so scary or triggering that we can't stay present and process what's happening, so our brain removes us from our conscious mind to enable us to escape the terror and survive. In a way, our urge to disconnect keeps us safe, helps us forget what happened, and allows us to keep going. It's adaptive, and though it can be helpful during a traumatizing event, it's not easy to control and can quickly become dysfunctional.

The definition of dissociation even in its simplest form, 'a break in how your mind handles information,' can make one feel like there is something wrong with them: we are broken. Somehow we are the ones that take on the shame for this fundamental mechanism that allowed some of us to survive. As a survivor I've been told by my therapist, doctor, etc., 'If you survived the abuse, you will survive healing from it.' Only they fail to realize that I wasn't even there mentally. I don't remember a lot of the details because I was dissociated. Most of the time I wasn't in my own body to experience the pain and trauma. I did not understand that what was happening would cause shame, hate, and disgust. I didn't even realize what was happening to me was even something 'bad.' It was like my body and my brain knew something was wrong, but not me, not little me.

CAN DISSOCIATION BE DIAGNOSED?

The first dissociative disorder recognized by the *DSM* is dissociative identity disorder (DID), which is characterized by a person having at least "two or more distinct personality states, which may be described in some cultures as an experience of possession."[2] These different personality states are often called "alters" since they can represent alternate parts of our character. This diagnosis used to be called multiple personality disorder because when an individual with DID shifts from one personality state to another, they can act like an entirely different person. This can be upsetting to both the person with DID and to those around them.

Along with these distinct personality states, those with DID also suffer from dissociative amnesia, not remembering what took place when they were in that other state, as well as dissociative fugues, which are when we don't remember key components of who we are and aren't able to recall how we got somewhere. This can be scary and make it difficult

40

for those with DID to function in their daily life.

In my experience, DID occurs because of intense trauma, where one part of ourselves cannot handle what's going on, and through continual dissociation and repression, we create other personalities to help us cope. This could mean that we have an alter that's more aggressive or protective of us, and possibly one that represents the part of us that feels like a hurt child. Everyone's alters are going to be different, depending on who they are and what they have been through, but we must get some professional help if we think this is something we struggle with. When I first looked into the treatment options for those with DID, I believed that integrating all of the personality states was the goal, and I released a video to that effect. My audience quickly let me know that that was not what's best for most people with DID, and integration can in many ways be just as traumatizing as their past experiences.

> Dissociation makes me feel floaty and lightheaded. At the very beginning, my heart feels like it's going really fast. I don't remember anything and I'm not able to focus on what's around me. Almost like I have no sense of what I'm doing, and I used to end up in places and not remember how I got there. It sometimes led me to do very risky things but not remembering I'd done them until I'd become less dissociated.

If we fight to merge all of their alters, we are not only forcing them to remember the past trauma, but also to remember all that they have done over the years. Being in a dissociative state can cause us to act in strange, hurtful, and dangerous ways; not remembering it is part of our self-preservation. Although we should slowly work together to process all that happened, and come to terms with what we do remember, that doesn't mean our alters will cease to exist. Without trying to completely eradicate them, we can instead get all of these personality states to work with one another in harmony instead of fighting with one another. I know this is hard to understand, but it's like these alters are our internal family, supporting us and helping us survive some of our toughest times. Without them, we can worry we won't survive or even know who we are; therefore, instead of trying to kick them all out, we have to get them to cooperate with one another, and therapy can help us do that.

The next dissociative disorder listed in the *DSM* is dissociative amnesia, and since we have already discussed this, I will keep this explanation short. Dissociative amnesia occurs with a traumatic or stressful experience and it's not like normal forgetting where we may forget where we parked our car. Those with dissociative amnesia won't remember important details about themselves or experiences they just had, even though that memory was already stored. It's as if it's just out of the reach of their conscious mind.

The interesting thing with this type of amnesia is that it is always reversible—meaning with the right help, they can remember it, whereas with other types of amnesia, the memory was never saved, and therefore cannot be recalled.

Finally, there is depersonalization/derealization disorder (DPDR) which, based on my experience, is the most common of all the dissociative disorders. Depersonalization is when we feel disconnected from ourselves. We can have a distorted sense of time, be unable to connect with our thoughts, feelings, or even our body. It can feel as though we are just watching ourselves go through our day, unable

> **"** Dissociating made me feel safe because it allowed me to escape from everything I was experiencing and then after the trauma had stopped it, protected me from remembering the things that hurt me for so long. It's almost like my brain tapped out and said, 'I need a break.' And dissociation was able to give me that. **"**

42

to have direct contact with what's going on in our head, which can be incredibly uncomfortable and scary. Many of my patients have said that when they are depersonalized, they feel numb, checked out, and disconnected, and even if they want to reengage, it's as if they are moving through mud and can't get there. I believe this happens because being in our body and witnessing everything that's happening is too much to manage; our brain's pulling us out allows us to keep doing what we need to do to survive.

Derealization, on the other hand, is when we feel disconnected from our environment. This means that it could feel as if we are in a fog or that everything in our world is out of focus and distorted. Many of my patients have explained this as feeling that they are in a dream or an alternate reality and everything around them doesn't feel real. When we have DPDR, we can experience disconnection from self or environment or both, yet even though we can feel completely disconnected from ourselves and our world, we still know where we are, who we are, and what we are doing.

I thought all people just didn't have many memories, like just a handful of 2- to 3-second clips and that was all, even when you were living it at the time. I also thought all people dissociated frequently, and everyone felt trapped in time. I thought everyone just felt like they were stuck at certain ages. Like my brain just forgot to grow beyond 17. But most of the time I feel like I am that fragile and hurting little girl, where everything and everyone around me is so very big and scary.

Another type of dissociation I want to touch on is called maladaptive daydreaming because, even though it's not in the *DSM*, it is common and important to understand. Maladaptive daydreaming is when our daydreams take over and we find ourselves preferring to spend time in that alternate reality instead of the one happening to us at the time. These are not normal daydreams where we imagine a perfect life or space out for a few minutes thinking about someone we have a crush on; maladaptive daydreams are used as coping skills and a way to avoid what's going on in the present. We can find ourselves having them if our current life is trauma ridden or overwhelming, or it could be our way to cope with any flashbacks or upsets that happen to us. We may never have learned how to deal with things in life, and so we created our escape to get us through.

Over the years, I have had patients tell me they will spend entire days daydreaming, not wanting to come back to reality or engage with their real life. That's why it's called "maladaptive"—meaning that it's not providing anything helpful to the person; instead, it's creating an entirely new problem. These daydreams can be very vivid, lifelike, and often have storylines or plots going, almost as if you are part of your own television show. Whereas we all can find ourselves drifting off to another place, or dreaming of a better time, we know how and when to return to reality; maladaptive daydreams get in the way of our ability to function. My patients who struggle with this also have difficulty getting to sleep, completing their work on time, and engaging in healthy relationships. Some have even been caught talking to themselves or moving oddly while daydreaming in public. Daydreaming in and of itself isn't harmful; however, if we find ourselves preferring the daydream over our real life, and spending hours engaging with it each day, it's time to reach out to a mental health professional who can assist us. Since it's often born out of trauma in our life, working to heal that wound should make the need to live in a daydream go away for good.

WHAT IF THOSE DIAGNOSES DON'T FIT MY ISSUE?

While those four dissociative disorders do help us to see the different ways it can manifest, I believe dissociation to be more of a spectrum. Depending on how triggered or overwhelmed we are, we will respond with different dissociative symptoms; I have even experienced this myself. A few years ago, I got into an argument with a good friend of mine, and if you know me, you know that I hate conflict; even the idea that someone might be upset with me can hijack my thoughts and ruin my day. Thinking back on this fight, I can recall being upset at her and her yelling at me for not wanting to go to a certain party, but all of the details are gone. Even as I sit here and try to put what happened to words, I can't. I know it happened to me, yet I can't remember what she said, or the events following it. I believe that's because her yelling pushed me into a short dissociative state. I couldn't handle the anger and upset, and so my brain let me step outside of the conversation for a bit. While that argument ended up ruining our friendship, I

Last month I experienced one of the worst cases of this. I was driving along the highway going to my house as I live a bit outside of the city. I have zero memory of what I was thinking about in this case, but all of a sudden I could feel everything moving slow and I started to get tunnel vision. I remember moving my head to the left as I passed the turn I was supposed to take, but I was unable to react to it. By the time my head came back to the front, I could see I was drifting off the highway and was now off the road in the dirt and grass, still driving forward. I still couldn't react. Then I saw I was headed straight for a power pole and was finally able to move the steering wheel, which caused me to go completely off the road and down the side, ultimately landing my vehicle in a shallow swamp. Once I had grabbed the wheel to react and try not to hit the pole, I snapped back into real time. I then spent the next 2 hours stuck in a swamp, waiting for a tow truck, while random people drove by staring at me. It was beyond embarrassing.

am somewhat thankful for my lack of memory during that time. It did allow me to get through it, not react, and get home safely. But if this happened to me all the time, I can see how it could be hurtful and scary, not to mention it could cause me to feel even more out of control and disconnected. The fact that I didn't get to choose whether my dissociation happened was disconcerting, and I do not want to feel like a passenger to my experience ever again, no matter how uncomfortable it may be.

It all comes down to our ability to manage the things life throws at us; if it's more than we can handle, we can find ourselves disconnected from our body or environment. That's why dissociation can accompany many situations, such as intense arguments, going through a divorce, or moving. It can also be a part of various mental illnesses, such as social anxiety, panic disorder, or PTSD. When our brain feels tapped and doesn't have the skills to deal with it all, it takes a break from reality and pulls us into a dissociative state.

HOW DO WE GET BACK WHEN DISSOCIATED?

Dissociation can feel like it comes out of nowhere: one minute we are present and able to focus, and all of a sudden we are caught up in a fog, watching ourselves from afar. It can be scary, upsetting, and embarrassing at times. The reason it can feel that it happens without warning is we haven't been able to figure out what triggers it. As we discussed, all five of our senses can trigger symptoms of PTSD; from a familiar smell to the sound and pitch of a voice. We can be going about our day, feeling fine, and then—*BAM*—we hear something that we connect to our trauma, and our brain pulls the ripcord, causing us to disconnect from everything.

Instead of feeling like an inactive participant in our dissociative symptoms, we need to take back control where we can, starting with our triggers. It's important for many reasons to identify and understand what upsets us, but when it comes to dissociation, we won't be able to prevent it from happening if we don't first know what causes it. Although what we remember of a dissociative episode may be a bit hazy or difficult to recall, the time just before it occurred is usually pretty clear. Think back to your last dissociative episode, and ask yourself the following questions to see whether it gives you any information as to what triggered it:

- Where were you? What were you doing?
- What did you feel, see, hear, taste, or smell?
- Who else was around you at the time?
- What is the last thing you remember?
- Have you dissociated in a similar situation before?
- Any idea how long it took for you to come back from the dissociation?

While that brief questionnaire isn't exhaustive, it does get us thinking about possible triggers and patterns. If there are specific areas or situations where we frequently dissociate, we can try to avoid them until we have the tools needed to prevent them from continuing to happen. It's not a complete fix, but it does give us a break from the disconnection and offer some much-needed information about our emotional limits.

Once we have identified a few common triggers, we then need to build up resources to help us better cope. Resources are just people, places, or things that can help support us when we begin to feel maxed out or that our brain is trying to pull us away. One of the most powerful resources is people in our life who know us well and to whom we feel connected. Now, I know that not everyone has someone in their life who knows about their trauma or mental health issues, but if you do, that person should be the first on your list of resources. Giving them a call when we are starting to feel overwhelmed can pull us back to reality and soothe our system. Texting can help, but phone calls or in-person meetings are best because there's no lag in responses, and hearing someone's voice and looking them in the eye can be much more powerful than a written message.

On that note, the next resource is our sight, and using our eyes to look at things that feel safe, pretty, and connected can help us more quickly regulate so that we don't dissociate. This can happen by looking at a loved one in the eyes, or even a pet. Any living being that we love and who feels safe can help us calm down; our amygdala—our brain's "fear center"—is always looking for a threat, and if we show it that nothing dangerous is going on, it may stop the stress response. We can also look at a waterfall or a flower, or really anything that is nonthreatening, and do our best to take in all of its details: What colors do we see? Is it textured or smooth? Hopefully, as we give ourselves time to take in all the visual information, we will feel that familiar pull of dissociation fade away.

One final visual example I want to share is one that I use in my office constantly: counting colors. If I feel my patient slipping away—maybe I have noticed their grip tighten, eye contact cease, and they stop talking midsentence—I will ask them how many items in the room have the color blue in them. Then, I move on to green, brown, or any other color I can think of until I can see they are a bit more relaxed and present. Prompting them to start noticing all that's around them and keep track of the number of items can be just enough to keep them from completely floating away from our session.

We want all of our resources to be soothing and help us, and another way we can accomplish that is through sucking and swallowing. Which I know sounds a bit odd, but it's why a crying baby is often calmed through being fed, and why many children suck their thumbs.[3] Our nervous system is wired from birth to pacify and connect us when we do this, and as an adult, we can mimic this experience by having hard candies on hand. The sucking and swallowing required when we enjoy a LifeSaver can be a quick resource to have with us at all times so that when we start to feel a bit overwhelmed or upset, we can just pop one in our mouth and let the natural action calm our nervous system down. Doing this can hold dissociation at bay and help us not get overwhelmed by whatever trigger we encounter.

I also want to mention that because sucking and swallowing are calming to us, those of us who have experienced trauma can also struggle with overeating or even binge eating disorder. It can be one of the only ways we are able to stay present and feel okay, but know other tools can help, and working with a mental health professional to process through that trauma will help us better manage our eating.

We can engage in resources that use our physical body, such as taking a hot shower or doing some movement, such as yoga or stretching. Even having a good friend or loved one rub our back or touch our arm to keep us present can help. One of my friends who struggles with DPDR used to ask me to sit next to her during large events so that I could rub her back or grab her arm every few minutes so that she wouldn't miss out on anything. This safe physical touch allowed her to stay grounded and present at a time when all her brain wanted to do was pull her away. If there is an action we can take that helps us be more aware of our body and the sensations we feel within it, let's try to do it.

Just make sure that these activities don't turn into a form of self-injury; they should simply help us stay in our body and feel how we feel. Too often, I have patients who will scald themselves in the shower or pinch themselves on their arms so hard they leave bruises. These physical movements are not intended to create pain or lead to use numbing out in other ways, so choose some that can be safely implemented.

I recognize how hard this can be. Dissociation happens for a reason, and it may have been our go-to escape our entire lives, so trying to do something that prevents that can feel impossible at times. But just as we learned in the last chapter, we can change our brain and get out of those unhealthy behavioral ruts; it just takes a conscious effort to pull our thoughts and behaviors away from what we used to do and into these new techniques. It's like learning to ride a bike: at first, we think about getting our feet on the pedals, going fast enough that we don't fall over, steering in the direction we want to go, and trying to balance. It can be overwhelming, and we will most likely fall a few times while we learn, but before we know it we will be hopping on that bike and riding away easily. It's the beginning that's the toughest when learning new things, so stick with it and know that, with practice, it will get easier.

Dissociation did have its pros and cons. I learned to use dissociation when it would benefit me. I used it when I didn't want to be present at doctor visits, the dentist's office, getting a tattoo, or even having my eyebrows waxed. Unfortunately, because I was so accustomed to using dissociation, I was unable to have a natural birth for my son. I could not stay present long enough to get through his birth and ended up having a C-section. Dissociation took that life experience away from me. I knew it was time to get this under control or it was going to completely control me.

WHAT IF I LIKE DISSOCIATING?

Many of my patients and viewers have asked why they need to stop dissociating if it makes them feel better and it's not hurting anyone, and while I understand that it can feel good at times, it hinders a lot of the work we try to do in therapy. Trauma therapy only works when we are present and in what many call our "resilient zone"—meaning that we haven't dissociated, and we aren't angry or in our fight-or-flight response; we are in our body, aware of what is being said and what we are saying. I could even go as far as saying we need to be in our resilient zone for any therapy to work, but we especially know this to be true when processing any past trauma. We previously talked about how trauma affects our brain and that when our amygdala senses a threat, it shuts down our prefrontal cortex and other parts involved in complex thought and decision-making. That allows for us to get out of any potentially harmful situation and survive, so it makes sense that we don't need critical thinking when we just need to run away from an ominous stranger in the alley. In the same way, if we are in a dissociative state and we cannot connect to our body, our thoughts feel all fuzzy, and we are completely zoned out, we aren't going to be able to do any therapeutic work. We can't recall our trauma memories, talk about how that made us feel, and come back next week to build from there. We may not even remember the last session!

Letting go of this comfortable coping skill is hard and we may want to let it take us away sometimes, but to stop our trauma memories from taking any more from us, we are going to have to find a way to stay present and work through it. I never said therapy was easy or that it wouldn't force us out of our comfort zone, but we need to trust that if we can push through the discomfort and fight for a better future, we will get there.

KEY TAKEAWAYS

- When something traumatizing happens to us, our brain can pull us out of our conscious mind so that we don't have to be present and experience the event. This removal from our consciousness, called dissociation, comes in many forms and levels of severity.

- The three main dissociative disorders listed in the *DSM* are dissociative identity disorder (DID), dissociative amnesia, and depersonalization/derealization (DPDR).

- There is also maladaptive daydreaming, which isn't in the *DSM* but is also common. This is when we would prefer to spend our time in our daydreams rather than our real life.

- To combat dissociation, we first have to identify the things that trigger it, and then build up some calming resources to help us stay present. These can include moving our body, sucking on hard candy, making eye contact with a loved one, and many more simple strategies.

- Staying present instead of checking out can be difficult, especially if we have been doing it for years, and that's why we will have to put some conscious effort into our resources and using them before letting our dissociation take us away.

- It is common for people to enjoy dissociation, but if we aren't able to manage it and stay present, trauma therapy—or any therapy—won't help us.

CHAPTER 5

WHAT IS REPEATED TRAUMA?

C-PTSD & HOW IT'S DIFFERENT

F or most of my patients and viewers, their trauma doesn't come from one experience; instead, it's spread over years or possibly a lifetime. While a diagnosis of PTSD does help describe what it can feel like to be traumatized, it falls short of explaining what being repeatedly hit with wave after wave of fear, pain, and terror can do to a person. We call this type of repeated trauma experience complex post-traumatic stress disorder (C-PTSD). C-PTSD is not included in the *DSM* but it is in the eleventh edition of the *International Classification of Diseases* (*ICD*-11). I only mention that because it's important to know that the symptoms have not been agreed upon or laid out for diagnostic purposes, but it is on the *ICD*'s list for its treatment to be coded and covered by insurance companies. In all honesty, it doesn't matter whether it's in any diagnostic manual or on any list of diseases and disorders; I know it exists because I have heard the stories and have seen it with my own eyes.

Again, when thinking about trauma, I don't want you to think only of our veterans. While many of them come back from war with C-PTSD, we also have first responders, abused children, people harmed by domestic violence, those who are in poverty, health-care workers, and many more. If we take the time to think about it, there are various ways we can be repeatedly subjected to traumatizing situations, and if we don't have the time or resources to process the traumas as they come, we can slowly be engulfed by them. Just as we discussed big and little Ts and how they can both lead to symptoms of PTSD, those who are continually hit with wave after wave of any traumatic situation never feel that they are on solid ground, or have a firm grip on their environment, and therefore can struggle to manage all that they feel. As a result, the symptoms of C-PTSD aren't limited to those of hypervigilance, struggling with flashbacks, and dissociation; it can go deeper than that, eroding our sense of self and ability to regulate our emotions. It's also important to know that some of the symptoms we will discuss are felt in PTSD, but not to the depth or severity that they are experienced in C-PTSD.

HOW IS C-PTSD DIFFERENT FROM PTSD?

Due to a lack of accredited symptomatology, those with C-PTSD are often misdiagnosed and not given proper treatment. Simply talking about how this differs from PTSD doesn't fully explain the experience, but this story from a viewer can hopefully help us understand:

> C-PTSD kind of feels like Jenga. Remembering difficult emotions or memories is like picking out a block and waiting for things to fall apart. Avoiding things so everything doesn't collapse around you and always being on high alert because "just in case something bad happens" and in every relationship, you're waiting for everything to fall or be scary because that's what you're used to. It's that constant worry that things aren't going to be right, so you have to check and recheck things which make it impossible to make decisions. Being hurt or expecting trauma is an everyday thing and there's no escaping how on edge you feel because of that. Sometimes you can come across as moody or having unstable emotions but in reality, it's just because your brain is trying to juggle so many thoughts and emotions relating to past experiences and trying to predict the

outcome of potential situations. And if the Jenga tower falls over, you know that it's your fault for trying to manage all of this.

I love that explanation and analogy—thinking of C-PTSD as a game of Jenga. With all the worry and fear swirling through our mind constantly, it's no wonder that the first differentiating symptom between it and PTSD is emotion regulation. As this viewer shared, "sometimes you can come across as moody or having unstable emotions . . ." Juggling all that's going on in our mind and being on high alert constantly is exhausting and difficult. If you think about it, being tired or overwhelmed can make us all more emotional and it can feel impossible to address life's ups and downs calmly and responsibly. We can come across as explosive or too sensitive when what's going on is that we are drowning in memories, worries, and trying to make sure we don't get hurt again.

Our difficulty regulating our emotions can take its toll on our relationships. On the one hand, we can lash out preemptively, thinking that we are protecting ourselves from further pain and suffering. We can also be short-tempered because we spend most of our day fighting off the thoughts, memories, and worries. Therefore, when someone asks us to help them out or gets upset about something we did, it can cause us to come unraveled. On the other hand, many of my viewers share how they isolate themselves as a way to deal with all they are going through, because it's easier to manage when there are fewer triggers. That way, we don't get asked how we are doing or why we aren't very talkative; we can just focus our energy on managing all of the thoughts and experiences that bombard us every day.

We discussed dissociative amnesia in the previous chapter, and why trauma memories can be fractured and difficult to fully recall; that still exists within C-PTSD; however, it's much more intense. Many of my patients and viewers struggle to remember any portion of their traumas, some sharing how experiencing yet another upsetting event pushes any memory they had out of reach entirely. I have

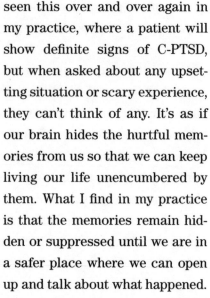

There's also a strong feeling that there is something wrong with you but you can't figure out why. The feeling like you are insane due to your overreactions to often small things. In some ways, learning about them makes you feel more unstable until you learn to handle those triggers.

seen this over and over again in my practice, where a patient will show definite signs of C-PTSD, but when asked about any upsetting situation or scary experience, they can't think of any. It's as if our brain hides the hurtful memories from us so that we can keep living our life unencumbered by them. What I find in my practice is that the memories remain hidden or suppressed until we are in a safer place where we can open up and talk about what happened. Once we are safe, the signs, symptoms, and bits of memory will bubble up and, in essence, urge us to process them.

C-PTSD can also make it hard for us to trust people. If we have been hurt repeatedly, possibly by multiple people, throughout our lifetime, it's going to be difficult for us to welcome anyone new into our life. Not to mention that because we have had such terrible and harmful relationships in the past, we can question our ability to vet people. This is where the effects of C-PTSD take the largest toll, by eroding our trust in ourselves and our abilities, and we can begin to think that something's wrong with us. Often wondering why we can't just be okay, move on, and live a normal life. We can even think that we did something to cause all of this.

Another differentiating component of C-PTSD is how we can have a distorted perception of our abuser or whoever harmed us; this could be a parent or other caretaker, a spouse, or even someone we considered a friend. Especially if the trauma occurred when we were young, it can be hard for us to understand how someone could say they love us while doing something hurtful. This can lead to us forming bonds with our abuser, wanting the attention they give us, and possibly even falling in love with them. I know this is hard to understand, but when we are young, we are primed for connection and attachment. If we are subjected to abuse during this time and told that this is what love, family, or attention looks like, we believe it. Psychologist Patrick Carnes calls this emotional connection a trauma bond, and it is believed that they are formed out of intense fear, terror, and a need to survive.[1]

Even if we don't bond with our abuser, we can try to make sense of it, thinking that maybe they really didn't mean to hurt us or perhaps we are the ones that caused it to happen. I cannot tell you how many times I have heard some version of "I didn't fight back after a while, so I think it's my fault that it kept happening." It can be hard for us to understand that if we can't fight back or get away from the situation, our only other option is to freeze until the trauma is over. This frozen state not only makes us feel helpless and scared, but it can also lead to a lot of shame and guilt. Just like that viewer shared earlier, "If the Jenga tower falls over, you know that it's your fault for trying to manage all of this." We take all the blame for the pain and hurt, unsure of whether our abuser deserves it. They can tell us they love us and that's how they show it, or possibly blame it on something we did as if we made them do it. If we repeatedly hear this for months or even years, it can be hard to not believe it or possibly wonder what's wrong with us.

All of these experiences and resulting symptoms can rob us of our sense of meaning in life.

> Trust is completely eroded into nothingness. And there are so many walls set up as a result of those traumatic incidents that everything appears fake. You start to question your reality and every interaction that you have. And interacting with every person is basically a new me, to the point where I have been having a huge crisis of identity, trying to pin down who I am.

Which as a therapist is scary, because meaning and hope are what help keep us motivated and alive. Whenever someone is losing hope or feels helpless against their struggles, suicidal thoughts are not far behind, and while I believe everyone can get better and life is worth living, I also understand why suicide feels like an option. When I asked my audience to share their stories, my inbox was flooded with messages like this one:

> People around me are over my shit. They think I am just lazy or not trying hard enough. They think that if I did more or just sucked it up and got on with things I would have a job and be out in the community. But most times I think they don't get just how bad it really is or how hard I am fighting. But it's hard with C-PTSD. And nightmares suck. Every night I am pounded with multiple nightmares of past traumas. Where I get trapped in these horrible scenarios, sometimes all of them at once, where I am hurt over and over again by these evil people and can't find any safety. Often jolted awake mid-scream and shaking, feeling so very small and fragile as I was back then. And some days because of how hard I am fighting my brain, the biggest achievement I can accomplish is getting out of bed. Most days it takes me hours to be able to pull my head out of that torture and convince myself that I am safe and grown. Some days it is as late as 7 or 8 pm before I can pull my head out of it, which is disheartening knowing that I have to do it all over again not long after. And the number of times that I have gotten in trouble for being rude or "trying to get attention" because some days I lose the ability to speak for a few hours. Where I can type and I can write to communicate, but I can't physically speak. And it takes me a while to regain my voice, but people around me just assume that I'm putting it on for attention.

It's stories like these that show just how important it is that we be understanding and compassionate toward those with C-PTSD, and why it can be so debilitating for those suffering. Being in traumatic situations over and over throughout our lives can take its toll on our emotional health and make it difficult for us to form healthy relationships. As we continue through the COVID-19 global pandemic, this understanding is even more vital since we will have essential workers emerge having been traumatized day after day, without a chance to vent or process it all. The less we judge and the more we listen, the better suited we will be to help them. As a therapist, it's a reminder to listen to my patients and let them teach me about their experience, so that we can work together toward treatment and healing.

STRUGGLING TO DEAL

When we feel that we can't seem to get our head above water, the traumas keep coming, and we are barely able to catch our breath, it's no wonder we try to find a way out of the pain. Coping with trauma isn't easy, and while dissociation can offer some relief, it's often not enough. That's why our brain gets creative when coming up with ways to numb the pain, or to help us feel alive again. Throughout my years in practice and online, I have heard them all; from over-spending to drinking, doing drugs, harming ourselves, and even using food and exercise to deal. Many of my patients whose trauma experiences revolve around sex can find themselves using sexual acts to cope, sharing how it made them feel they were taking their power back. Here's an example from a viewer about all of the ways she tried to cope:

My experiences with C-PTSD all started with being exposed to childhood sexual abuse that lasted for a couple of years. At a young age, I wasn't prepared for a life that would consist of recurring sexual trauma. Throughout my early teens, I struggled with anorexia and hated my body, it never felt like my own, I was very introverted, I had issues with trust and was emotionally withdrawn. This shifted during my later teens into alcohol and substance abuse and becoming sexually promiscuous without any emotions attached.

In many ways, we try to grab hold of anything that will give us a break from our pain and suffering. These various coping skills can change over time, depending on what we need or how we feel. One of the most common unhealthy coping skills for C-PTSD is self-injury. And before you jump to any conclusions, no this isn't for attention or a suicide attempt. Self-injury is often a way to physically show all of the emotional pain we are experiencing. It can be done to numb out from all we feel, or even be a way to create an event where we have to tend to our own wounds, in essence physically caring for ourselves because we don't know how to do so emotionally. I have also had many patients tell me that it's a way to let out all they feel, as if the physical hurt releases the emotional pain.

Since self-injury doesn't help us process all we have been through or get more connected with ourselves and how we feel, its relief is short-lived. The act of self-injuring can lead us to have a whole slew of other issues as a result. For example, when we self-injure, it's usually done in secret and there are shame and embarrassment around the action. We can fear anyone finding out because they might think we are crazy or not understand why we do it. Too often, I hear of people being put into the psychiatric hospital because a family member or even mental health professional didn't understand or know how to treat them. I don't want to downplay the potential for infection and other complications stemming from self-injurious behavior, but once the injury has been properly cared for, it's important to understand the emotional side of it and what it means to the person who is engaging in that behavior. That's why my advice is to listen and seek to understand someone's experience before jumping to any conclusions. Doing so can save all of us any additional pain and ensure that the proper support and treatment are given.

Another type of coping skill I see concerning C-PTSD is eating disorders. I know you are probably wondering what food and exercise have to do with trauma, and in all honesty, they aren't related at all. The reasons we use eating disorder behaviors to cope are in some ways the same reasons many use self-injury: We want to numb out and not think about the real pain we are experiencing. Eating disorders allow us to focus on and control the one thing we can, our body. Putting all of our focus and energy into what we eat or don't eat can be a welcome distraction from the flashbacks, waves of emotions, and worry about the future. To explain this with more clarity, here's a story from another viewer:

Everything in my life felt out of control. I was having a hard year at work, I couldn't fix my mom's issues no matter how hard I tried, I couldn't keep my family together as we were falling apart, but I could control myself, and I could most definitely control my eating and my exercise. I developed an eating disorder in college, but I have been in recovery for several years, feeling healthier and so much more free than I had during those years in college. However, when the family stress and trauma came into my life, I found myself becoming more food-obsessed. I started to track my food again, measure everything I put into my body, and exercise daily, too much exercise for the number of calories I was consuming . . . I believe that because of this, my eating disorder has returned because it makes me feel like I finally have control over something in my life, and nobody can take it away from me. Nobody can take away this power I have, and that gives me a sense of security back in my life. The more I control the amount of food that goes into my body, and the more I exercise, the more I feel like the world isn't spinning me around anymore. When I eat less, I feel calm. When I run, I feel calm.

I do want to mention that not all eating disorders cause you to lose weight, and they don't happen only to women. If you were already imagining a young girl who looks emaciated, I want you to think again. My eating disorder patients have been every age imaginable, and at least half of them struggle with binge eating, not restricting. An eating disorder occurs when we use food as a way to cope with how we feel, and almost all of our thoughts each day are food-focused. That's it. Sure, we can get caught up in the symptoms and which eating disorder diagnosis fits those symptoms, but I don't care about the diagnosis. What I care about is figuring out why the eating disorder exists in the first place. What was going on in our life when food became such a focus? When did we start overeating? Undereating? Or overexercising? You would be surprised how many of my patients will tell me they have no idea why they struggle so much with food, and that their life is fairly normal and happy. But just a few sessions later, we have uncovered how their father used to drink too much and hit their mom, or that they were bullied for four years in school. It's normal for us to stuff down any traumas and upsets so we can keep going, but it will come out one way or another; in many cases unprocessed trauma will erupt in eating disorder behaviors.

There are various ways we can try to cope with a trauma-filled life, but the last ones I am going to discuss here are alcohol and drugs. I feel that we hear about this one the most: how people who have been through a traumatizing situation drink or do drugs as a way to dumb out and forget that it happened, and it makes sense. If we are inebriated, we truly cannot think straight, focus, or process all we have been through. We can just zone out and relax; that is, until the high or alcohol wears off and then we are back where we didn't want to be, with all of our thoughts and feelings rushing back. We can get caught up in this cycle of numb out, sober up, and do it all over again.

In the wake of COVID-19, the market research firm Nielsen reported that alcohol sales were up 27 percent, and though many argue that it was because people were not drinking out at restaurants and bars, I think there is more to it.[2] Many people live alone, are feeling stressed and worried, not to mention Alcoholics Anonymous (AA) and Narcotics Anonymous (NA) meetings aren't taking place in person anymore. Needless to say, the spike in sales is a bit alarming. Too often, we fight to find a way to ignore all we feel instead of working to process it. As our world continues to be subjected to traumatic experiences, we must take note of all the ways we try to numb out instead of tap in and validate how we feel. I know it's uncomfortable, and we aren't always ready for it, but if we keep ignoring it and covering it up, it will only fester and cause us more pain.

KEY TAKEAWAYS

- Complex post-traumatic stress disorder (C-PTSD) happens when we are traumatized repeatedly.

- The symptoms of C-PTSD that are not included in the PTSD diagnostic criteria are difficulty regulating emotion, issues in our relationships, struggle to recall anything about the traumatic experiences, inability to trust others or ourselves, distorted perceptions of our abuser or perpetrator, and struggling to find meaning in life.

- Due to the COVID-19 pandemic, it's likely that most of us will experience some form of trauma. Noting what symptoms of trauma affect us and finding ways to talk about all we are experiencing, whether with a therapist or friend, can help us overcome this together.

- Numbing out from the pain of C-PTSD is common and can be done through self-injurious actions, engaging in eating disorder behaviors, or abusing drugs and alcohol, to name a few.

CHAPTER 6

ARE WE SURE IT'S C-PTSD?

Too often, C-PTSD is misdiagnosed and mistreated. Since we are not taught about it in school and the *DSM* isn't any help, most mental health professionals have to learn about it through colleagues or by treating patients with it, if they learn about it at all. This lack of information and understanding has led many patients to be seen for a short time, feel misunderstood, and then referred out, seeing three or four therapists a year while trying to find someone who will help them process it all. This can be disheartening, invalidating, and painful. I believe this all stems from a lack of understanding and the fact that many of the symptoms of C-PTSD overlap with those of borderline personality disorder (BPD).

BPD is a very misunderstood mental illness and is characterized by an intense fear of abandonment, a pattern of unstable relationships, and impulsive behaviors, often born out of trauma. As far as the *DSM* is concerned, someone with BPD shows, "A pervasive pattern of instability of interpersonal relationships, self-image, and affects, a marked impulsivity, beginning by early adulthood and present in a variety of contexts."[1] Already you can see how this could overlap with some of the symptoms of C-PTSD, at least when it comes to difficulty in relationships. However, BPD is a much more pervasive diagnosis; the criteria go on to cover nine other symptoms or behaviors; to be diagnosed with BPD, we must have at least five of them.

The first criterion and one of the ways I differentiate BPD from C-PTSD is "frantic efforts to avoid real or imagined abandonment."[2]

When we have BPD, we can believe deep down that we are unlovable and bad and therefore are not deserving of love or affection. Instead of allowing someone to leave us, which would be too painful for us to endure, we lash out and may try to leave them first. This can be hard for others to deal with, they can think we are hateful, easily upset, or overly emotional. The real reason we do this is to protect ourselves; we can't trust that someone will always be there for us, or be trustworthy, so we strike first. Many of my patients have shared how they often lash out to see how people react, in hopes that those individuals will apologize and tell them how important they are, but too often, this outburst ends up harming the relationship and, in turn, the person with BPD.

Although this criterion can in some ways look like those of C-PTSD because we can be emotional and our emotions can feel out of control at times, the big difference is why we feel that way. Do our emotions feel out of control because we are dealing with so many flashbacks, nightmares, and trying to predict another trauma? Or is it because we are so sensitive to any perceived loss or abandonment? Of course, to find this out many of us will have to see a mental health professional, but once we think about it, I am sure we can figure out which diagnosis fits us best.

Next up, we have "a pattern of unstable and intense interpersonal relationships characterized by alternating between extremes of idealization and devaluation."[3] This one could be a bit tricky because those of us with C-PTSD can struggle in our relationships, making them unstable or intense; however, the last portion about alternating between extremes is purely a BPD thing. If we can go from loving someone to hating their guts within minutes, it's more likely BPD instead of C-PTSD. When it's C-PTSD, our relationships can become unstable because we are dealing with so much pain and turmoil internally that we can struggle to trust, communicate, and have patience with those around us. We don't idealize someone one moment only to think they are the worst person to ever walk this earth the next.

Moving along, the next criterion is hard to tease out and could be why so many people with C-PTSD are misdiagnosed as having BPD. This symptom is "identity disturbance: markedly and persistently unstable self-image or sense of self."[4] When it comes to BPD, this expresses itself through shifting goals, career plans, who we want as friends, and what our core values are. Since many of those with BPD can believe something is wrong with them or that they are bad in some way, they can quickly switch between being needy and clingy to strong and assertive. This is done as a way to connect and get support, but also protect them from the perceived threat or upset. This happens in some ways with those who have C-PTSD, since they are constantly on the lookout for another potential traumatic situation; however, the big difference is when it's C-PTSD, we are trying to figure out who we are in this dangerous world. When it's BPD, we are trying to get connection and attachment by being whoever we think we need to be. It's more like we chameleon ourselves to start or continue a relationship.

The next criterion is impulsivity, and one main area of overlap between BPD and C-PTSD. The *DSM* states that we must show "impulsivity in at least two areas that are potentially self-damaging."[5] These are such things as overspending, being hypersexual, or binge eating. The *DSM* does not include self-injury in this section, but I believe it should be there since that kind of behavior is impulsive and urge driven. With regard to C-PTSD, we can be impulsive in some ways because our mind is focused on so many other things, and binge eating does happen as a way to cope with the pain of the trauma. It does present more as being reckless, which can be a form of self-destructive behavior, and that's why I would say that this is one portion of the two diagnoses that are the same, but remember you have to have five of these symptoms to be diagnosed with BPD, so they are still very different.

The fifth criterion is yet another reason many of us with C-PTSD are diagnosed with BPD. These symptoms are "recurrent suicidal behavior, gestures, or threats, or self-mutilating behavior."[6] Self-injurious behavior can happen for various reasons; however, it's only in the *DSM* under the diagnosis of BPD. And just as a note, the *DSM*-5 did mention "non-suicidal self-injury" as a *Condition for Further Study* but it hasn't been included yet. Therefore, if we go to see a therapist or other mental health professional and let them know that sometimes we harm ourselves when we are feeling bad, they could automatically diagnose us with BPD. Now, I would hope that they would spend more time with us, ask questions, and look for other symptoms of BPD, but I know that's not always the case.

When it comes to the difference between C-PTSD and BPD concerning this, there may not be any. I know that many of my BPD patients have used suicide and self-injury as a way to test their relationships, to get some extra support and care they were craving, or to try to end all of the pain they feel; however, that's not always the case. The way I distinguish between the two is to ask questions about why they self-injured: Did it have anything to do with a relationship? Possibly it was done to express an upset from an argument or breakup? If that's the case, then it's most likely related to BPD; if it was done to manage all of the anxiety, panic, or body memories, then it's caused by C-PTSD.

Next, we have "affective instability due to a marked reactivity in mood,"[7] and you can see again how this could look a lot like C-PTSD. After all, when we have been traumatized over and over again, we can be easily irritated, upset, and struggle to control our moods. However, when this is related to C-PTSD, we will struggle with emotion regulation as we process through all the trauma, and that could last months or even years. When this symptom comes from BPD, these outbursts or reactivity only last for a few hours and on the rarest occasion a few days.

Another symptom of BPD is "chronic feelings of emptiness."[8] In BPD, this can be due to our struggles in relationships and constant worry that we will be abandoned. Many even report being easily bored, which can lead them into acting impulsively or lashing out. However, in C-PTSD, it's more common to have a negative outlook on life and struggle to look for reasons that the traumas occurred, but again it's not related to abandonment or our relationships. The upset and detachment we feel is focused on the traumas and trying to ensure we don't get hurt again.

The second-to-last symptom is "inappropriate, intense anger or difficulty controlling anger."[9] In BPD, I believe this comes from our belief that something is wrong with us or we are just bad, and that's why everyone will leave us. While those thoughts and beliefs aren't true, it can lead to angry outbursts because we are just so full of shame and upset. Those with C-PTSD can lash out and be easily angered, it's not usually as severe as those with BPD. The difference between BPD and C-PTSD regarding these criteria can be hard to discern, and again, shows us why these two diagnoses are so often mistaken for the other. That's why all mental health professionals must spend time with their patients; listen to them; ask questions to figure out where the urge, upset, or other symptoms are coming from; and then decide which diagnosis is best.

The final criterion can easily be linked to BPD and C-PTSD, and it is "transient, stress-related paranoid ideation or severe dissociative symptoms."[10] We have already discussed how dissociation is part of PTSD as a whole, and a way for our brain to cope with all of the pain and trauma. Those who have been traumatized can also be paranoid that it will happen again, like this clip from an earlier example from one of my viewers:

It's that constant worry that things aren't going to be right so you have to check and recheck things which make it impossible to make decisions. Being hurt or expecting trauma is an everyday thing and there's no escaping how on edge you feel because of that.

The real difference in how these symptoms are expressed in BPD versus C-PTSD is that those with BPD feel this way due to real or imagined abandonment, and those with C-PTSD have these in response to trauma triggers in their environment. Again, it can be hard to spot the difference, but by having a conversation about when the symptoms began or digging into what triggered the sensation, we should be able to figure out which diagnosis explains it best.

As you can see, there are many overlapping or similar symptoms between these two diagnoses, and that's why many people get misdiagnosed with BPD when it should be PTSD, and vice versa. It's also important to know that many people meet the criteria for both diagnoses. A recent study found that 24 percent of those with PTSD also had BPD[11] and 30 percent of those with BPD also had PTSD.[12] They used the PTSD diagnosis in these studies because, as I shared earlier, C-PTSD isn't in the *DSM* and doesn't have any clear diagnostic criteria.

Another diagnosis that is often misrepresented as C-PTSD is bipolar disorder; however, the differences between these two are not as nuanced as with the previous one. While there are two types of bipolar disorder and many ways it can present, the important thing to know about bipolar disorder is that it's episodic. That means people with bipolar disorder of any kind go through episodes of elevated energy and feeling really good about themselves as well as experience periods of feeling really low and depressed. C-PTSD is not episodic; unfortunately, we feel the symptoms of it all the time. Therefore, the easiest way to discern between these two diagnoses is to track the symptoms and see how long they last. I often work on timelines of the symptoms with my patients to see how often they come up, what triggers them, and how long they last. This helps us better prepare for and manage the symptoms.

Overall, when diagnosing and treating someone with C-PTSD, it's important to rule out other diagnoses that could look and feel very similar, to ensure we know what we are working on. Even though a diagnosis isn't everything, we do need to understand the symptoms that are bothering us so that when we reach out for help, others know what to assist us with. To check that you completely understand what C-PTSD is and is not, here is a quick questionnaire:

- Have you been traumatized multiple times in your life?
- Have you repeatedly witnessed someone else experience a traumatic event? One in which you feared for their safety?
- Do you worry more days than not about another trauma happening to you or those you love?
- Are you constantly assessing your environment for any signs of a perpetrator or unsafe situation?
- Do you struggle to manage all you feel, and think you overreact to some of the smallest things?
- Have you ever used self-injury, sex, eating, or alcohol or drugs to deal with how you feel?
- Do you find it almost impossible to trust people?

If you answered yes to the first or second question and to at least one other question, you could be suffering from C-PTSD. The next helpful step is to reach out to a mental health professional in your area or online who knows how to treat PTSD and understands the nuances of C-PTSD. And yes, it is perfectly okay to ask them about these disorders as relates to their training before making an appointment with them. We want to make sure we find the right person to help guide us on our path to recovery, because we can and will get better.

WHY DO I KEEP BEING TRAUMATIZED?

One of the most common questions I get about C-PTSD is "Why do I keep getting hurt? Am I doing something to lure bad people into my life?" and I understand their concern. If it seems that every relationship or situation we get into leads to us being hurt, we can start to question ourselves and what we are putting out there into the world. If we consider the symptoms of C-PTSD, we can see some ways they could be working against us.

One of the first symptoms is that of the freeze state. If we were in a traumatizing situation and fighting or fleeing weren't options, we could go into a state of freeze. Freezing can be a helpful stress response because it can prevent us from potentially causing ourselves more harm; for instance, if we fought back knowing an abuser is much stronger, we could end up with broken bones or possibly be killed. Therefore, in many ways, our freeze state can save us. However, when we are repeatedly in situations in which we cannot fight or flee, and instead have to go into our freeze state, we can slowly develop learned helplessness—meaning that because we have tried to deal with everything that's happened to us, yet no matter how hard we try we don't succeed, our automatic response can be to give up.[13] This can hurt us in future situations because even if we could get away or fight back, our brain automatically goes into freeze, rendering us helpless and increasing the likelihood that we are hurt again.

On the flip side, many of us who grew up in constant trauma or stress can become so used to the environment it creates that we look for relationships or situations that feel just like it. In the same way people joke about dating someone just like your mother or father, many of us with abusive parents can in essence do the same thing and find a person that is just like our past abuser. Being in this continuous state of stress can also lead us to overlook it in our regular life. We could be walking down a dark alley late at night and not think anything of it because we are used to feeling at risk or on edge, whereas someone without C-PTSD wouldn't be comfortable and would most likely run out of that situation or not put themselves in it to begin with.

The final symptom of C-PTSD that can lead to us being hurt again is our distorted perception of ourselves and our perpetrator. Being traumatized multiple times can cause us to question ourselves and our ability to properly assess other people. Furthermore, if we formed a trauma bond with our abuser, we can feel even more confused and unsure of ourselves. This can cause us to get into unhealthy relationships and be talked into doing risky things. If we don't think we can trust our intuition because it hasn't served us well in the past, we can look outward to others and hope that they will make the right decisions for us. However, this can put us in more traumatizing situations.

HOW CAN I STOP IT FROM HAPPENING AGAIN?

I don't want to leave you thinking that if you have been traumatized more than once, there isn't anything you can do to stop it from continuing to happen, because that is not the truth. There are many things we can do to fight against those symptoms that can hurt us, and lean into the ones that keep us safe. The first thing you can do is to find a mental health professional who understands C-PTSD. I know that's obvious, but it's really important to find someone you can trust, and since trust can be hard to offer in our daily lives, a therapist is a great place to start. Then, you can use them to vet other people, letting them know what was said, how you felt, and together you can decide how to proceed.

Next, be a detective. Not as if you are trying to solve a crime; more of a detective of yourself and your past situations. If you can, look back on the last relationship you were in that was hurtful. Did you have any inkling that it was going to be abusive? Were there any early signs that they weren't a good person? Maybe you have friends or family who can weigh in on these situations; you could ask them whether they sensed anything before the traumatizing event. I know memory can be hard here; that's why I made getting a therapist the first tip, but family and long-term friends can help out where our memory isn't as sharp. Being a detective also means keeping track of our symptoms and feelings. This can be hard at first, but trust me, with practice it gets easier. Making a list of the symptoms I discussed in this chapter can help. Maybe write them down on one side of a piece of paper and note things that you did that day that fell into each category. And if feelings are hard to name, you can simply search online for a "feelings chart" and tons of forms with lists of feeling words will pop up and you can download or print them off.

My final tip is to take your time. Too often, we rush into relationships or situations without giving ourselves time to get to know people, letting them meet other people in our life, and having a chance to see them in various environments. If we take our time, fight any urges to be impulsive, and check in with those we know and trust, it's less likely that we will find ourselves in yet another hurtful situation. Also keep in mind that anyone who doesn't respect our time frame and wants to rush us into decisions isn't worth our time anyway.

C-PTSD can be difficult to deal with and we can feel like we keep getting hit with wave after wave of trauma, but with proper understanding, support, and hard work, it does get better. We can heal and go on to live a life free from the symptoms and pain that have been holding us back all this time.

KEY TAKEAWAYS

- C-PTSD is often misdiagnosed as borderline personality disorder (BPD) or bipolar disorder. That's why it's important to see a mental health professional who understands the differences.

- Those with C-PTSD can be more likely to be traumatized again, for many reasons. First, we can feel helpless to stop it from happening again. Second, we can be so used to living in a traumatic or stressful environment that we seek it out. Finally, our distorted perception of ourselves and our perpetrators can make it hard for us to know who's good or bad.

- We can prevent trauma from happening again by seeking the support of a trauma therapist, using our past traumatic situations to help us better prepare and protect ourselves, and taking our time getting to know people first.

CHAPTER 7

WHAT ARE THE 4 ATTACHMENT STYLES?

WHY TRAUMA IS ROOTED IN CHILDHOOD

My first job working as a therapist was at a free clinic in North Hollywood. We saw mostly court-mandated cases: some struggling with addiction, many active gang members, and a lot of children affected by their parents' divorce. My first therapy patient was a ten-year-old girl named Isabella. She was having a hard time at school, unable to keep up with her homework, and getting into fights with her peers. Her teachers recommended she see a therapist and a psychiatrist to assess whether she needed to be placed in a special needs classroom for disruptive children. Isabella was quiet at first, struggled to make eye contact, and only wanted to color or play with the wooden dolls I had in my office. As a new therapist, I was worried that I would never get through to her or get her to share with me what was going on, but after seeing her every week for two months, she started to open up. She began incorporating this plastic dinosaur toy from another toy bin into her therapy play. She made the dinosaur hit one of her wooden dolls over and over again, yelling at it, while she hid the other doll behind her. I asked Isabella who the dinosaur was and she just shook her head, brought back out the other wooden doll, and continued to play with the two dolls again as if nothing had happened. I wasn't sure why such a simple question had shut her down, and I worried that I had done something wrong or hurt our new therapeutic relationship. Whatever had happened, I needed to find out more about it and do better next time, so I went to my supervisor.

At this time, I was still an intern and therefore had weekly supervision with a licensed therapist to help guide me when I felt lost and ensure I was offering quality care. His advice was to wait until she brought out the dinosaur again and ask some things about the other characters since she didn't feel safe enough to talk about the dinosaur. I took some notes based on what he said and waited for our next appointment together. She kept playing without the dinosaur for the next few weeks, but finally, it made another appearance, and this time I had a new way to approach the subject. I asked who the doll was that she hid behind her and asked her whether that doll was safe and okay. She still shook her head, not able to talk about the scenario she was demonstrating through play, so I asked whether she wanted to color or draw instead. She loved that idea and helped me get out all the crayons and paper. While we colored, I asked many questions about what she was drawing, who her best friend at school was, and tried to get to know her better. It's important to let you know just how slow work with children can be, especially those who have been traumatized. They don't trust easily, nor do they know how to tell you what's going on. Maybe they don't have the words or have been told that if they do say something, they or someone they love will be hurt. Isabella and I colored for another month or two before I was able to find out that the doll she hid while the dinosaur hurt the other doll was her, and that she had to hide to be kept safe. Yes! I was finally getting somewhere!

Over the next few months, I came to learn that it was her mother who was being hit by her boyfriend, and Isabella would hide in the closet in her room when he came over or when he raised his voice. He had hit her a few times in the past, and that's why she had decided to hide in her closet. An unfortunate part of my job is having to report situations like this to Child Protective Services, the governmental agency that helps protect children. As a therapist, I am a mandated reporter—meaning that I am legally bound to report any child, elder, or dependent adult abuse that I hear about or see in my practice. Even though I talked with the mother and let her know that I had to report it, she never brought Isabella back to see me, and I often think about her and hope that she is doing okay. I know I did what was right, but when seeing children, it can be hard because they aren't in complete control of their life and who's allowed in it. As someone who got into this line of work to help people heal, I struggle with situations like this and often wonder whether I could have handled it better. I was a brand-new therapist, and while I did ask my supervisor to ensure what I was doing was correct, should I have done something differently? Did I inadvertently cause Isabella more harm than good? I may never know.

IS CHILDHOOD TRAUMA COMMON?

Unfortunately, Isabella's story isn't an anomaly. Before the age of sixteen, two-thirds of children report experiencing at least one traumatic event.[1] Which means that most of us have faced at least one upsetting and terrifying situation, and while we know that with proper support and care we can process the trauma and be okay, the younger we are, the less likely it is that we have any emotional understanding or ability to deal with it. These earlier life traumas can shape who we are and who we decide to get into relationships with. For many years, we didn't know how to assess for these early life traumas or what effect they could have on us as we get older. That all changed in 1998 when the Centers for Disease Control and Prevention (CDC) and Kaiser Permanente published their Adverse Childhood Experiences (ACEs) Study based on seventeen thousand adult patients and how their childhood trauma exposure affected their mental and physical health later in life.[2] This groundbreaking study proved that there was a connection between ACEs and future health concerns—meaning that the more traumatic childhood experiences we had, the more health concerns we will have as we age.

They based their findings off of ten ACEs: emotional, physical, and sexual abuse, physical or emotional neglect, domestic violence, parental mental illness, substance dependence, incarceration, and parental separation or divorce. These ten ACEs do not include things that come from our environment, such as bullying, poverty, or racism, and because those situations can have a detrimental effect on us, many clinicians have begun to add them to their assessments as well. While the demographic information of those included in the study are not the most diverse, it's still important to note that even with the participants being almost 75 percent white, about half were sixty years of age or older, and 39 percent of them had completed college, almost two-thirds of those studied reported at least one ACE. Also, one in eight reported four or more ACEs.[3]

When I first heard about this study, I immediately wanted to take it myself to see whether I had any ACEs, and I would assume that you are no different, so here is an adapted ACEs questionnaire:[4]

- Before your eighteenth birthday, did a parent or other adult in the household often or very often swear at you, insult you, put you down, or humiliate you? Or act in a way that made you afraid that you might be physically hurt?
- Before your eighteenth birthday, did a parent or other adult in the household often or very often push, grab, slap, or throw something at you? Or ever hit you so hard that you had marks or were injured?
- Before your eighteenth birthday, did an adult or person at least five years older than you ever touch or fondle you or have you touch their body in a sexual way? Or attempt or actually have oral, anal, or vaginal intercourse with you?

score of 4 or more were two and a half times more likely to have hepatitis, chronic obstructive pulmonary disease (COPD), and many other health concerns.[5] Now, you could look at this data and think that it's obvious that those who were traumatized when they were young would be more likely to drink, smoke, and engage in risky behavior, but it's much more than that. Even if we don't engage in any risky behavior, those of us with high ACE scores are still more likely to develop health issues. You might be wondering why that is, and the truth lies in our stress response. When we get scared or stressed, our body sends the signal to our brain to release stress hormones, such as adrenaline and cortisol, and we enter our fight/flight/freeze response. This makes our heart pump faster, our airways open so we can breathe better, and our pupils dilate so we can see more clearly. Our body readies itself for action. This stress response helps keep us alive and helps us run away from danger or fight back against an attacker. However, it's not meant to be engaged for long periods, and if our environment keeps us held in that stress response day after day, it's no longer lifesaving, it's hurting and hindering us.

In the ACEs Study, they call this type of stress "toxic stress" and it affects our brain development. It can decrease the response from the reward center in our brain (the nucleus accumbens), which is responsible for sending a signal alerting our midbrain that we have been rewarded and tells it to release more dopamine, making us feel amazing. When this part of our brain isn't as responsive, we can feel more depressed or struggle to find enjoyment in our lives. This could also be what leads those of us with a high ACE score to turn to drugs or alcohol to get that rewarded feeling or high. Elevated ACE scores can also affect the amygdala, or what I like to call the fire alarm in our brain. It's responsible for initiating our fear response, and if it's activated too frequently, it can become enlarged and lead to symptoms of hypervigilance. It can also lead to us being so used to feeling on edge or at risk that we struggle to know what's dangerous or not. The prefrontal cortex is our brain's control center and decision-maker and is vital for learning. I like to think of our prefrontal cortex as the adult part of our brain. It can take into consideration all of the information, manage our emotions about it, and help us calmly make decisions. When we have a high ACE score, this part of our brain is impaired, which can make us more impulsive, struggle to plan, and have difficulty creating goals for ourselves.

As you navigate your answers to that ACE questionnaire, try not to minimize what you have been through. It's so common that we think, "Well, that only happened when he had a bad day," or "I know she didn't mean it." Take into consideration just how you felt at the time as a child, and whether you felt unsafe or worried that your parent or caregiver was going to lose control and hurt you; count that as an ACE. Going back to what we discussed in the second chapter, being traumatized has more to do with whether we thought we or someone we love was in real danger and less to do with what happened. The ACE questionnaire continually mentions "often or very often" when asking us if something happened to us when we were young, which leads me to believe that most of the ACEs are examples of experiences that could cause us to have C-PTSD.

Having a high ACE score doesn't mean that things can't get better or that we are doomed to have health issues for the rest of our lives. Dr. Stephen Porges researched people being held in their stress response for long periods and tried to find out what we could do to help calm ourselves down and feel better. What he came up with was the polyvagal theory.[6] In short, while studying our vagus nerve, Dr. Porges identified a third type of nervous system response (we used to think we only had two: activating or calming); this third response that he identified was the social engagement system. What he found was instead of our nervous system being either more activated and less calm or calmer and less activated, it could do a little of both. We could be activated through social interaction while also calming our system down. It's the safety we find in true connection with others that helps us manage and more quickly calm the stress response. This means that the best way to overcome the hypervigilance or stress we can feel from our adverse childhood events is to have safe, nurturing relationships. Making time for these connections is the true antidote to our stress response and any upset we have experienced.

WHY IS IT SO HARD TO CONNECT TO OTHERS?

We learned through the ACEs Study that having these adverse childhood events can lead to more health concerns later in life. Our emotional development starts in our first year of life when we attach to our primary caregiver, and in the psychology world, we call this first connection our attachment style.

The theory of attachment styles was first researched in the 1950s by British psychologist John Bowlby.[7] After working for many years at the Child Guidance Clinic in London, he had become fixated on understanding the distress and upset children experience when separated from their primary caregiver. I use the term *primary caregiver* because not all children are raised by a parent. In some families and cultures, it's more common for a grandparent or aunt to raise the children or even a nanny. Whoever we count on to tend to our basic needs is considered our primary caregiver and the person with whom we attach to. Bowlby defined attachment as a "lasting psychological connectedness between human beings." And he believed attachment to be all or nothing—meaning that we either have a healthy attachment or we don't. However, this definition and all-or-nothing approach didn't explain children who would cling to a parent and then want nothing to do with them. There was more to it than being attached or not, and that's where psychologist Mary Ainsworth came in.

In the 1970s, Ainsworth devised a standardized assessment for attachment behaviors in children called the Strange Situation

Classification (SSC). In short, she observed children as they were put through eight different scenarios where the child, its mother, and a stranger was introduced, separated, and reunited. Each scenario lasted three minutes, and she scored the children's behavior based on four criteria: (1) Proximity and contact seeking, (2) Contact maintaining, (3) Avoidance of proximity and contact, and (4) Resistance to contact and comforting.[8] After observing one hundred children, Ainsworth identified three main attachment styles: secure, insecure-avoidant, and insecure-ambivalent.[9] This was the first study to support and expand on John Bowlby's theory of attachment, and in 1990 two researchers, Mary Main and Judith Solomon, used Ainsworth's SSC to discover a fourth attachment style that they called "disorganized."[10]

Throughout Mary Ainsworth's studies, the majority of children were securely attached to their primary caregiver. When a child has this type of attachment, they will feel easily soothed and safe when with their primary caregiver. If they are distressed, they will turn toward their caregiver, or seek them out in some way. This attachment is formed when a child knows they can count on their caregiver to be there for them when they cry, soothe them, and care for them. They will use this secure attachment as a safe base from which they can explore all that's around them.

The next observed attachment style is insecure-avoidant. Children with this style do not attach to their caregivers because they don't feel they can count on them. This usually means that their primary caregiver either hasn't been there for them when they needed it or has been rejecting or dismissive of their needs altogether. This could be in response to a parent who was emotionally or physically neglectful of their child, or if we go back to the fourth question from the ACEs Study, "Before your eighteenth birthday, did you often or very often feel that no one in your family loved you or thought you were important or special? Or your family didn't look out for each other, feel close to each other, or support each other?" If any of that is happening to us in our first few years of life, it is going to be hard for us to feel safe to navigate the world. We can believe that something is wrong with us, or that we are unworthy of love and attention. We may not know who to trust or think that we can't trust anyone. In Ainsworth's study, when a child is in distress and has this type of attachment, they will not seek contact with their primary attachment figure. They won't even show a preference between their primary caregiver and a stranger. Again, this is because they aren't sure who will help them or what adult figure will offer support and security.

To further explain this type of attachment I want to share part of a story from one of my viewers:

My whole childhood, as far back as I remember, had been being told by my father that I was a mistake, a financial drain on them and that he and my mother would be happier if I wasn't there. My mother would just stand there and say nothing—she would kind of treat me like I wasn't there, saying nothing negative or positive, just nothing. I think that because of this I was a quiet and withdrawn child. I remember crying a lot because I was so confused all the time. My parents hated or ignored me for reasons I didn't know. I had no idea why the kids at school hated me so much, I always tried to be nice, until after a while I just stopped talking. I never understood why no adult would ever help me. My parents would have people come over and play cards (I had to stay in my room) and I would always hear about how having me was a mistake and if it wasn't for me they would have bought a nicer house, and that I cried about everything for no reason . . .

The confusion caused by neglect and emotional abuse can make it hard for us to enter into new relationships and we can question

the validity of any relationship we get into. Even if someone contin-
uously tells us we are important and that they love us, we can still
worry that they will leave or hurt us, which could be too much for us
to take. I have had many patients with this style of attachment, and
the majority refuse to entertain the idea of romantic relationships or
any close friendships; the risk just felt too high.

The third style of attachment Ainsworth observed was insecure-
ambivalent. Children with this type of attachment tend to be clingy
and needy of their caregiver, but when the caregiver comes to their
aid, they reject them and are not easily soothed. This is usually in
response to their primary caregiver not being predictable in their
support. Perhaps they are comforting and soothing one minute only
to be hurtful and abusive the next. While the child will want to be
soothed by their caregiver, they aren't sure whether the caregiver
can give them what they need. That's why even if their parents come
to comfort them, they don't soothe easily; they are still waiting to
make sure they are safe.

I have always referred to this style as the anxious type because
children who are raised feeling like they are walking on eggshells,
not sure whether their parents will be comforting or hurtful, grow
up to have symptoms of anxiety. These can be caregivers with mental illnesses that cause mood swings or struggle with substance
abuse or even two caregivers who have drastically different parenting styles. Again, you can tie some of these issues back to the ACE
questionnaire and see how devastating this can be to a child. When
we are growing up and developing, and we learn that sometimes
our caregiver is loving and comforting, but other times they aren't,
we try to figure out why. Because we can't know or understand the
real reason behind the hurtful behaviors, we assume it's something
we did. Many of my patients with this style of attachment are over-
achievers and perfectionists because they grew up believing that if

they did everything just right, they would get the love and attention they so desperately needed.

The final style of attachment is disorganized. Children with this type of attachment will show a confusing mix of attachment behaviors and may even appear to be confused or disoriented. They believe that this attachment style is caused by inconsistency from their caregivers—meaning that a parent may be soothing and helpful, but also fear-inducing and hurtful. While you may be thinking that that sounds a lot like the insecure-ambivalent style, a disorganized person doesn't have any pattern to their behavior. It's not them clinging to their caregiver and then not being easily soothed; instead, they may not want anything to do with their caregiver, or other times cry until the caregiver comes and holds them and then are soothed easily. In essence, they aren't sure what they feel or whether they can count on their caregiver. This is usually born out of abuse, where there aren't any other caregivers around, and the child associates them with love and support and also fear and pain. Therefore, they oscillate between secure responses and insecure-avoidant ones. I believe this wasn't observed in Mary Ainsworth's SSC study because in the three minutes of observation, she probably only saw one type of response from the children, and didn't get to see them move between the two attachment styles.

WHAT CAN UNHEALTHY ATTACHMENT LEAD TO?

You may be wondering what attachment styles have to do with trauma, but the two are closely connected. Our first few years of life are key to developing a strong sense of self, feeling confident in ourselves and our abilities, and believing that we are safe to go out into the world. In essence, our primary relationships help shape who we will become and what future relationships we will have. It's like a blueprint for connection and communication. If we are hurt, neglected, or upset constantly as a child, we may look for those same things in our life moving forward—meaning that those of us who grew up with loving, predictable, and comforting parents have a secure attachment and are more likely to get into other relationships that offer those same things. On the other hand, if we had caregivers who were unpredictable, abusive, or emotionally neglectful we can seek that out too—which can put us in more potentially traumatizing situations as we navigate life.

If we experienced trauma within our first few years of life, it can take therapy and a lot of work to get us to believe that the world is a safe place and that we have a right to be in it. It can be hard for us to think we are loveable, important, or that people care, and that can cause us a lot of shame. Shame isn't something that's talked about very often, and I believe it's because most people don't know what it is, not to mention that it's an uncomfortable feeling to acknowledge. In short, shame isn't just feeling guilty or upset about a situation; shame runs deeper than that. When someone is covered in shame, they truly believe that something is wrong with them, or that they are defective in some way. Embarrassment could be considered a mild form of shame, but embarrassment comes about due to a specific situation, while shame encompasses our entire self and all that we are. In cases where people are traumatized many times throughout their life, especially if it started when they were children, it's common to wonder whether they are doing something to cause continued pain. To further illustrate this, I want to share another viewer's story:

The trauma that I endured as a child has forever changed how I look at the world and would eventually give me the diagnosis of C-PTSD. Although I view myself as a healthy adult now, it took me many years of hard work, therapy, and EMDR to get here. During my healing from trauma, I learned just how much C-PTSD shaped me. I became aware of the hidden shame that caused a devastating self-hatred. I believed that if I continued getting hurt, I must be the one causing it.

When working in therapy to heal from trauma, it's the shame that's the most difficult to overcome. I've even had patients tell me that they deserve to have hurtful or bad relationships, some even getting into abusive situations and sharing how they believe it's the best they can do. It's heartbreaking and at the root of why we can feel so stuck in our trauma. If we honestly believe that something is wrong with us, and therefore we deserve to be treated poorly, why would we all of a sudden think that it could get better? We wouldn't. However, because the pain or other symptoms of trauma are often too much to carry alone, we reach out for help, and even though it is hard work, we can heal.

I also want to share how and why attachment issues can make their way into our therapy appointments because, too often, my patients feel even more shame about their struggles with our therapeutic relationship. Just know that our relationship with our therapist can often reflect our past relationships, and we can treat our therapist just as we did the person from our past. In a way, this is our brain trying to work through past trauma or upset, or we may not know of another way to have a relationship. Either way, it's normal to oscillate between feeling connected to our therapist and wanting to push them away so we don't get hurt. It can be confusing to be in a relationship with someone where they care about you, how you are doing, and want to help you feel better. This consistency and clear communication can feel foreign and scary, so give yourself time to get used to it and let your therapist know about these feelings as they come up. Our therapists cannot read our mind, so the more information we can give them, the better. That way, they can help us figure out where these thoughts and urges are coming from and help us heal.

HOW CAN I HEAL FROM CHILDHOOD TRAUMA?

When our trauma is rooted in childhood, reparenting (also called inner child work) must be part of our therapeutic work, and no I don't mean that we have to have our friend or spouse act like our parent: that's not how this works. This therapeutic technique doesn't involve our parents or caregivers at all and is completed in therapy with the sole purpose of healing ourselves from our past trauma. Reparenting is when we mentally take ourselves back to the time when the traumas occurred and work to heal that part of ourselves. For many years I have used letters to help start this process, asking my patients to write a letter to their child self, and having their child self write letters back. It can help us to feel heard and understood and give a voice to ourselves at a time when we didn't think we had one. The goal of reparenting is to give ourselves the love and comfort we needed as a child so that we can have a healthy and happy life now. In a way, we are rewriting our blueprint for life and our relationships, since the one we were given was unhealthy and traumatizing.

When doing this work, I often have my patients come up with some loving parental phrases that they wish they heard. These could be things like "you are important to me" or "I love you just as you are" or "I see you." Making a point of writing these things in the letter to our child self can help us give ourselves what we needed back then. And I know this all kind of sounds crazy and maybe a little woo-woo for you, but I promise, it works. We cannot go out into the world hoping that someone else will fix what happened to us in the past; what that does is force us to rely on other people to heal us and give us what we need, and other people are out of our control. If we try to use other people to help us heal, we will only be left feeling more alone or hurt when they let us down or do something upsetting. They are only human, they have their faults, and they cannot be responsible for our healing. Therefore, the best and only person we can count on to heal us is ourselves, and of course, a good therapist can help guide us along as we work through it.

We can also reparent by doing the things we wished our parents had done, such as take us to that amusement park or go on that trip. It could even be simple things, such as cleaning a wound on our knee or taking care of ourselves when we are sick. We can do these things without outside help—sure, it would have been better if our caregivers had done it when we were growing up, but it's great that we have the tools to do it for ourselves now. Try your best to focus on that and know that it will be strange and uncomfortable at first, but it does get easier and more healing with time. If you have a tough time coming up with things to do, your therapist can help you think of some, while also giving you a chance to talk out the times you were hurt, let down, or upset by the shortcomings of your caregivers. Just know that with time and professional support, we can heal that hurt child inside of ourselves.

Another way we can heal from any attachment issues we have is to be more mindful of our emotions and discomfort in relationships. It's very common to not know how we feel in certain situations, but it's much easier to notice or remember a time when we felt uncomfortable. By paying attention to these things, we will be better able to identify people or situations that trigger our attachment issues. Maybe it's the fear that someone will leave or let us down, or perhaps it's letting anyone get too close; whatever it is, being able to identify it is more than half the battle.

Once we have a better idea of what's triggering us, we can then work to better regulate our emotions so that we don't lash out or isolate. Following are a few dialectical behavior therapy (DBT) techniques that I find helpful.

Checking the Facts

The first DBT technique is Checking the Facts.[11] When we are acting out of a past upset, we may overreact in the present and even feel embarrassed about this reaction later. Checking the Facts forces us to slow our reaction time down by noticing what emotion or event triggered the response. Then, we check in to see whether we are making assumptions or interpreting something without having all the information. Too often we don't have any evidence, other than our past experience, to support what we think is going to happen. Taking the time to double-check our thought process and any assumptions we may have made can prevent us from lashing out and hurting ourselves or an important relationship. Finally, we note whether our initial reaction was in line with what we assumed to be true, or what we have evidence to support as truth. Overall, this ensures that we aren't acting a certain way because of something that happened to us at another time; instead, we are slowing our reaction down, considering the facts, and deciding how to respond.

Opposite Action

Another DBT technique that can help is Opposite Action.[12] Whenever we are triggered or upset, there are a bunch of emotions or urges that can come along with it. We can feel angry and want to shout, punch, or run away. If we are hurt, we may want to cry, stop talking, and isolate. These automatic emotional responses aren't always commensurate with what happened and can be coming from past experience. Using Opposite Action allows us to see we have a choice in how we respond and can help change our painful emotions into more helpful ones. It can also help stop us from lashing out and causing ourselves more pain and upset. An example of how to properly use Opposite Action would be that if my best friend cancels on me last minute, I might feel upset, sad, and as if I am not important enough. I could want to dodge her calls or texts, not reschedule our get-together, and spend the rest of my day crying. Opposite Action would mean that I would push myself to engage in conversation with her, tell her that I am disappointed and let her explain the late cancellation, and even reschedule. I know this is difficult, but we always have a choice as to how we respond to life's ups and downs; we just have to create the space and time for those choices. Taking back the control from our emotions is empowering and gives us a chance to grow and thrive.

ABCs PLEASE

The final DBT skill focuses on ways that we can reduce our emotional vulnerability—meaning that by using these techniques we are taking care of our basic needs so we aren't so easily thrown off by an upsetting situation. This skill is called ABCs PLEASE,[13] and it works like this:

A: Accumulate positive emotions. One of the easiest ways to do this is to take some time each day to do things we enjoy doing or to focus on things we are grateful for. This helps us gather some positive emotions so we feel better and are better able to manage any upsets that come our way.

B: Build mastery. By doing things we enjoy and getting better at them, we not only accumulate some positive emotions, but we start to feel more confident and competent in life. These tasks could be things like cooking, playing an instrument, doing some art, riding a bike, organizing our space, etc. The more regularly we do these things, the better we will feel and the easier it will be for us to weather any emotional discomfort.

C: Cope ahead. Having a plan in place for when we feel down or upset is key, that way we are prepared for whatever life throws our way. We can "cope ahead" by putting together a list of things we can do that make us feel good, people we can call who are supportive and loving, or some things we can do to distract ourselves if other things don't help. Putting together this plan will ensure that when we feel overwhelmed and want to lash out, we have something else to do until we are more clearheaded and able to make a thoughtful choice.

PL: Physical illness. When we are sick, we aren't at our best; therefore, we have to make sure we are taking care of ourselves. If we are sick, we need to rest or possibly make an appointment to see a doctor. This also means we have to take any medication as prescribed and take a few moments every few days to check in on how we are feeling physically.

E: Eating regularly balanced meals. Waiting until we are starving is not only bad for our body, it's also bad for our ability to regulate our emotions. The term *hangry* (a combination of the words *hungry* and *angry*) exists for a reason, so make sure you are eating a variety of foods every 3 to 4 hours to ensure you have energy throughout your day.

A: Avoid mood-altering drugs. It can feel good to numb out from all we feel through nonprescribed drugs or alcohol, but remember that those substances don't make anything better. Mood-altering drugs can cause us to be even more emotionally vulnerable then we were before. Consider only drinking in moderation and avoiding all nonprescribed drugs.

S: Sleep! Not getting enough sleep can make us more irritable, easily upset, and run by our emotions. Not to mention how hard it can be to focus or concentrate when we are tired, which can make remembering our emotion regulation skills even more difficult. Do your best to sleep and wake around the same time each day and allow for at least 8 hours of sleep each night.

E: Exercise! I know the word *exercise* can be triggering for many of us, making us think of slogging away in a gym day after day, but that's not what I am talking about. Making time in our life for exercise means that we do what we can each day. Some days, that may be stretching and then walking for 15 minutes; other days, that may mean we take an hour-long yoga class. My goal for my patients is to get them to a place where they can do some form of exercise for 30 minutes, 3 to 4 times a week. Exercise releases endorphins and other mood-boosting chemicals, which can make us feel better, and better able to manage anything life throws at us.

Overall, we must take the time to care for our basic needs each day. I know that sounds pretty simple, but on those days when we aren't our best, it can be hard to do. Sometimes, all we can accomplish is getting up to go to the bathroom, and that's why we have to check in with ourselves and use our ABCs PLEASE skills before we allow our thoughts and choices to be driven by emotion. When we have a past filled with ACEs and failed caregivers, it can take time to learn how to recognize and manage all we may feel; it's as though we are building a new muscle we didn't even know we had. Be patient with yourself as you try out these new tools, and as always it's a process, not perfection.

KEY TAKEAWAYS

- Childhood trauma is very common, occurring in two-thirds of children aged 16 and younger.
- The CDC-Kaiser ACEs Study helps us better understand childhood trauma and how to identify ACEs early on.
- The higher our ACE score, the more likely it is that we will have health complications later in life.
- Safe, nurturing relationships are the key to overcoming our ACEs.
- There are four styles of attachment: secure, insecure-avoidant, insecure-ambivalent, and disorganized.
- We can overcome our ACEs and attachment issues with the help of a trauma therapist and using reparenting techniques. The DBT skills Check the Facts, Opposite Action, and ABCs PLEASE also help us better manage our emotions along the way.
- Healing from childhood trauma is hard but completely possible.

CHAPTER 8

CAN TRAUMA BE PASSED DOWN?

TRANSGENERATIONAL TRAUMA
AND ITS LASTING EFFECTS

D uring the Cold War, which lasted for roughly forty-four years, the Communist Party took over Czechoslovakia, and in 1948, it built three parallel electrified fences along its border with Germany; this electric fence was called the Iron Curtain. It was heavily patrolled by armed guards, and close to five hundred people were killed attempting to escape. This fence was taken down when the Cold War ended in 1991; however, the local red deer still refuse to cross the area where it once stood. In 2015, Czech biologist Marco Heurich and his colleagues published their findings from a seven-year study where they followed three hundred red deer using a tracking collar and found that even though the average life span of a red deer is only fifteen years, they were still affected by a barrier that existed over twenty-four years ago. The researchers believe it's because the mother deer take their fawns near the old border but never allow them to cross it, therefore passing on the fear of the area and belief that it's not safe to roam into German territory. The researchers also followed deer on the German side and came to the same conclusions.[1]

Although these studies were conducted on red deer, not humans, it still tells us that trauma can be passed down from generation to generation, and possibly onto other people in our lives. In many ways, trauma can act like a virus, moving from one person to another until all those around us feel some of the effects. We call this type of trauma transmission transgenerational or intergenerational trauma, and it was first noticed in the children of those who survived the Holocaust. In 1966, psychologists in Canada reported that the grandchildren of Holocaust survivors represented a majority of their referrals, citing that they were three times more likely than others to seek mental health support from their clinics.[2]

WHO CAN BE AFFECTED BY TRANSGENERATIONAL TRAUMA?

This type of trauma doesn't only happen to those in the Jewish community, however; we can find examples of transgenerational trauma everywhere we look. A brief search online returns thousands of research studies conducted in different parts of the world all with the goal of explaining why those who haven't been in or witnessed a traumatic situation themselves are still experiencing PTSD symptoms. Some lived through the Holodomor genocide in Ukraine, which claimed millions of innocent lives through forced starvation, not to mention the Native American populations being forced onto reservations back in 1851. These two examples happened on other sides of the world from the Holocaust, and yet many Ukrainian and Native Americans struggle with similar trauma-based coping strategies, such as binge eating, substance abuse, distrust of the surrounding communities, isolation, and hostility.[3] It doesn't matter where we live or what trauma we were exposed to; we are all human, and the effects of terror can last for generations.

We also see transgenerational trauma in the Black community stemming from both slavery and racial inequality. I was just watching a video online the other day where a Black father shared how he taught his children to interact with the police. He asks his daughter to share what he taught her, and she states her name and then with her hands up says, "I am eight years old, I am unarmed, and I have nothing that would hurt you." The fact that we live in a society where this father has to teach his eight-year-old what to say, should she encounter the police and they have a prejudice that could put her in danger, is terribly sad. I do not doubt that this can affect the emotional growth and development of a child. Imagine being taught and told from birth that you are different and people will unfairly judge you because of it. I believe all of these scenarios are traumas that we cannot help but be personally affected by.

There is also transgenerational trauma within the immigrant community, due to discrimination, not being able to immigrate together as families, and possibly living in poverty until they can find better work. This can take mothers or fathers away from their children at a young age as they make the move to build a better life for themselves and their family, which we know can affect a child's attachment. Here is a story from a close friend of mine sharing her experience with this:

I was left to be raised by my aunt and grandmother at a young age so that my mom could make a better life for both of us by migrating to the United States. When I migrated to be reunited with my mom as a teenager, I found out that my mom was left by my grandmother to be raised by an aunt and also to start working at the young age of 11. Later on, as I grew up, I learned that my grandmother had also been left as a very young child to be raised by an aunt because her mother died when she was just five years old.

Looking back at this pattern, it makes so much sense why I struggle with attachment and constantly worry people will leave me. Sometimes even fearing to let people get close, worrying that I will get too attached. For generations, my family has engaged in this system of traumatic abandonment, and although I am still dealing with the ramifications of it, it has also shaped who I am today, and is a constant reminder that I can overcome any obstacle life throws at me.

The list of who can be affected by transgenerational trauma has no end, from those living in poverty to refugees, women, people in the LGBTQ+ community, and everyone in between. If someone in our family has been traumatized, we could feel the effects in our own life, and that's why we must recognize PTSD symptoms early on and get professional help quickly. While it can be tricky finding a therapist who understands trauma as well as what it can be like for a person of color, refugee, or immigrant, they are out there. Refining our search to include therapists who say they specialize in trauma; or are certified in such trauma therapies as EMDR, schema therapy, or somatic experiencing; as well as asking them upfront about their background and experience can ensure we find someone who is a good fit. In addition, I believe that being educated on these important issues should be a requirement for licensure and added to all health-care-based educational programs. When people are brave enough to reach out, I would like to know that someone caring and competent is there to help.

WHY DOES TRANSGENERATIONAL TRAUMA KEEP BEING PASSED DOWN?

We learn a lot about ourselves and the world around us from our parents or caregivers, and if they are dealing with trauma and upset, how can they not pass it off onto their children? We have already learned just how many symptoms come along with PTSD, and how difficult it can be to manage them. If we are trying to parent at the same time, it's like trying to teach someone to downhill ski while learning it yourself.

Transgenerational trauma continues to be passed down for two main reasons; first, most of us don't realize we are struggling with it because we've never known another way; and second, healing from trauma is hard work. Not knowing we were traumatized or that we could do things differently is by far the most devastating to our children, because there's no attempt to do better. I see this every day in my practice: a parent comes in angry or upset that their child is acting out, claiming that something is wrong with the child and they need me to fix it. It takes all of my strength to calmly explain to them that although a child may suffer from a mental illness, it's often exacerbated by what's going on at school or in the home. I have even had parents not come back after I gave them feedback on their style of discipline, offering some other ways that could be better for their child; this is part of the reason I began only seeing adults in my private practice. Too often, the parents would stand in the way of any tools or tips that could help their children. In essence, they tied my hands and then wondered why their child wasn't getting any better. It was exhausting and heartbreaking.

When parents are not able to recognize that they do play a role in their child's physical and emotional development, it's even more difficult for the child to get the help that they need. This is what leads to generations of shared trauma and patterns of unhealthy behavior. It could be the reason that for three generations the women in one family all married alcoholics, or it could be to blame for an entire family's fear of flying. The sooner we accept that through nature and nurture we affect our children, the sooner we can start working toward a better future.

We all know that healing from any trauma is difficult, and we are also aware that parenting is hard and trying at times. Putting those two things together can make not passing down our upsets feel impossible.

Having an awareness of our mental health issues and any traumas we have endured is a giant step in the right direction. I am constantly being asked by parents how they can talk to their children about emotions, mental illness, and any difficulties they are going through. This is a sign that we have a lot of great parents out there who are just trying to do their best for their children. Since I am sure

> I feel like I look at transgenerational trauma differently because I have a 7-year-old and she shows signs of having been traumatized despite not having anything traumatic happen to her. She is a normal happy little girl, but she still jumps as I do at loud noises and she gets very upset whenever we talk about my family despite never meeting them and she hates being alone at night, just like I did at her age.
>
> I feel like part of the reason she displays these behaviors is because I do/did and as far as I'm aware, so did my mum. Most of what children learn is from their parents. I didn't learn love or compassion from my parents so with her it's us figuring it out. When trauma and abuse have been passed through generations, it often feels like you are fighting a losing battle because it's going to happen no matter what you do. You and your family have been in pain for so long that you don't know what to do. I guess the only thing you can count on is that environment also has a big impact on a child so breaking away from the cycle (like me and my daughter did), it hopefully won't be destined for her like it was for me. I just need to make sure what happened to me doesn't change her worldview.

that those parents aren't alone, let's dig into some of the questions I see on a regular basis.

WHAT DO I SAY IF MY CHILD ASKS ME WHY I'M SAD?

Too often, we try to hide our feelings and upsets from our children. Trust me when I tell you that they already know all about it. They just don't know how to approach us or ask what's going on. Whenever a child asks about our emotional state, we must lean into it and let them know it's okay to ask. Start by looking them in the eye, thanking them for checking in on you, and then explain what's going on in a very simple manner. For example, let's say you just got some bad news at work and didn't get the raise you wanted. It's completely fine to tell your child that you thought you were going to get an award at work and make more money, but you just found out you didn't and that makes you feel sad. Children aren't as judgmental as we are, so let's use that to our advantage. They just want to know what's going on and whether they had anything to do with us being upset. Setting the story straight in a short and easy-to-understand way will prevent them from internalizing any of our stuff.

WHAT IF I TAKE OUT MY
ANGER ON MY KID?

Trust me, you are not alone in this, and this is a judgment-free zone. Everyone does it from time to time. We have a bad day followed by a worse evening, and we yell at our kids. We can have a lot of things going on: We could be stressed about money, going through a divorce, or not feeling well. No matter what the cause, we owe our child an apology. I know that sounds strange, but yes, we can apologize to our children when we take out our issues on them. Along with my answer to the first question, tell them what's going on that's upset you, and that you are sorry you yelled at them. Be honest about why you did it and ask them whether they understand and accept your apology. This is not a time to offer a gift or treat, even though we may want to make it up to them. The only way we can make it up to them is by trying harder next time. We want any apology we offer to be met with emotional support, conversation, and understanding, not just purchased goods or presents.

CAN I SHARE TOO
MUCH WITH MY KIDS?

Since we discussed how helpful it can be to talk with our children about how we are feeling, and why we may have lashed out at them, I think it's also important that we discuss boundaries around these conversations. Our children should only know about things that affect them and their relationship with us—meaning that if we are emotional at home, we should explain briefly why, but we do not need to get into all the details with them. Our children are not our close friends and engaging in that sort of relationship with them is extremely unhealthy. If we want to vent about all that's going on, we should reach out to a close friend or find a therapist in our area. Talking to our children as if they are equals or adults can cause them to act like one and in turn rob them of their right to continue acting like a child. In the therapy world, we call this being a parentified child, and that's not something we want to pass down either. Overall, we want to talk openly with our children about emotions, upsets, and our relationship with them, so that they feel comfortable to do the same. We just want to be careful that we don't think of them as our emotional support and someone we come to with all of our problems. That's not a healthy parent-child relationship.

DOES MY FAMILY HAVE
TRANSGENERATIONAL TRAUMA?

If you are still wondering if you experienced transgenerational trauma or not, here is a story that hopefully will shed some light:

> I sat here thinking if any of my mental health issues could have been passed down to me. I thought about how my mom used to

say, "Sometimes, I just want to drive off this bridge," but it was said more for means of getting what she wanted and to make me feel bad for her. So, I thought no, I don't think that has anything to do with my stuff, so I wasn't going to respond. Until BAM!!! I think I've discovered something interesting that wasn't recognized before. I am certain my dad had PTSD and didn't realize it. As a child, he battled polio not once, but twice. He spent a good bit of time in the Shriners Hospital. I asked him one day what that was like and he said it was really hard to make friends and then watch them die. He said he had a best friend who would go to the IV treatment room with him and they would always sit next to each other. And then one day, they rolled him in, but not his friend. That was how he found out [his friend] didn't make it. Fast-forward 50 or so years later, and my sister and I were taking him in for his first chemotherapy appointment. My job was to stay with him while they hooked him up and my sister's job was to do all of the paperwork. They had him in a room sitting in those big chairs (like the ones when you give blood) and I was just talking to him while we were waiting for them to come hook him up. I looked over at him, and he was frozen. I said "Daddy" several times and he didn't move. Then I said "Paul" and he looked to both sides, then to me, and started to cry. I was 23 years old and this was the only time I ever saw him cry, followed by a complete nervous breakdown. He kept begging me to take him home, and I helped get him out of there. He ended up not having chemo that day. We had to take him later that week to the hospital where they could give it to him in a room by himself.

That night, when it was just me and him at home, I asked him, "What happened today? I've never seen you cry before or panic like that." He said, "When I saw all of those people lined up beside me for chemo, I saw all of the kids in the Shriners Hospital all over again and I felt like I was back there. I just can't be there again. It took me too long to erase those memories."

My dad was never diagnosed with PTSD, but I think he had it. I'm not saying that it was necessarily "passed" down to me, but his trauma reaction is the same as the one I am dealing with now; hiding it from everyone, FREEZE, and holding back tears until you can't anymore. So maybe? If that's possible, it passed to me from my father.

There are so many ways we can be traumatized in our life, from growing up in poverty to losing a close friend when we were young. If you are still curious whether trauma could have been passed down to you, here is a quick questionnaire.

- Has a parent or close family member ever talked about a dark or difficult time in their life?
- Are there certain topics that are off-limits to ever bring up? Or were you told to stop asking about those things as a child?
- Has a parent or close family member shared any experiences of trauma (e.g., going to war, dealing with illness, abuse, etc.)?
- Have you experienced some of the PTSD-like symptoms but don't have any memory of being in a traumatizing situation?
- Can you recall any behaviors by your parents or grandparents that in retrospect could be a trauma coping skill (e.g., hoarding food, alcoholism, not going out at night, etc.)?
- Were there certain rules or behaviors in your house that your friends thought were odd or that you never saw in anyone else's house?

If you answered yes to more than one of these questions, your family may be experiencing transgenerational trauma. While it can be difficult to break these cycles, with personal awareness and professional help, we can overcome it.

DOES TRAUMA CHANGE OUR DNA?

We know that we can pass down our trauma responses onto our children and they in turn can act like they have been traumatized as well, but does this passing down of trauma change our DNA? Researchers have been trying to answer this question for years, but they have already stumbled upon some interesting findings. In a 2013 study led by Brian Dias at the Emory University School of Medicine, they found that a fear of a certain smell could be passed down to our children and even our grandchildren. They conducted this study on mice, and after conditioning a group of male mice to fear the smell of cherry blossoms by giving them an electric shock when the scent was released, they bred them with a group of female mice. What they found was that the children and grandchildren of these male mice were jumpier and showed signs of fear when the scent was released. They compared these mice to those whose fathers weren't conditioned to fear the smell, and there was a stark contrast. They also tried adding a neutral scent and all the mice acted normally—meaning that it was only the cherry blossom smell that put them on edge, which could only have come from their father or grandfather's experience.[4]

While they still believe we need more robust data to prove that fear of a specific scent can be passed down from one generation to the next, researchers do agree that trauma does not change our DNA. However, it does change the way our DNA is read or interpreted, otherwise known as our epigenetics. Epigenetics are markers on top of our DNA that tell us how our DNA should be read, and they are highly influenced by our environment—meaning that if we have been physically abused for years, our epigenetics will want the parts of our DNA responsible for our fight/flight/freeze response to be clearly read, and possibly overdevelop certain areas that could help keep us safe. These epigenetic markers are passed down to our children and they can cause us to have symptoms of PTSD even if we have never been exposed to trauma.[5] For years, researchers argued whether it was nature or nurture, but now we know that our environment shapes how our genes are interpreted.

Knowing that trauma can change our epigenetic markers can be validating and helpful, but it can also be upsetting. If our epigenetics are altered, can they be altered back? Further research does show that just as hurtful things in our environment can change the way our DNA is interpreted, nurturing and helpful things can too. They have found that nurturing relationships can change our epigenetic markers for the better—meaning that having a loving and nurturing person in our life can undo some of the damage the trauma has caused.[6] As a therapist, this is what I love to learn about, because we can't go back in time and undo the trauma or work to forget all of the pain we endured, but we can increase the number of nurturing relationships we have and the amount of time we spend in them. These connections will not only calm our nervous system down, but also help realign our epigenetic markers so that it's not only reading the parts of our DNA assigned to our stress response, for example, but also those parts responsible for deep connection and overall health.

CAN WE PASS TRAUMA TO PEOPLE OTHER THAN OUR CHILDREN?

Unfortunately, trauma isn't just shared with our relatives, but also to those around us. We can pick up behaviors, reactions, and beliefs from those we are in close relationships with, and therefore be affected by one another's trauma. We know that our environment can change our epigenetic markers, so it's no wonder we can pass our trauma on to our friends, roommates, and colleagues as well. I believe this shared trauma is exacerbated by social media because it allows us to be closely connected to more people, increasing the likelihood of us encountering a trauma response. It can also make it more likely that we see something terrifying or upsetting as well.

In May 2020, a video was released showing a police officer in Minneapolis taking George Floyd into custody and kneeling on his neck for almost nine minutes until he was killed. People all over the world had access to that video and everyone I know has watched it at least once. It is horrific, intensely upsetting, and difficult to put words to. I believe anyone who watched that video shared in that trauma, and although the full effects of it have yet to be discussed, we have seen an outcry from the masses for police reform and justice for the victim.

All of this connection can bring us together, help us learn from one another, and work together toward common goals, but it can also spread trauma like wildfire through our world. Now more than ever, we are a global society; we travel around the world with ease and communicate with people anywhere with the touch of a button. All of this connectivity has both helped and hindered us toward the end of 2019 with the emergence of COVID-19. From the first known cases in November 2019 to March 2020, the entire world went into a government-forced lockdown, shutting down any nonessential businesses, closing borders, and enacting stay-at-home orders. I still remember being so confused, scared, and unsure of what was happening. We had had outbreaks in the past with the bird flu and Ebola, but businesses had never been forced to close and we hadn't been forced into staying home.

Wearing a mask, while necessary, makes it hard for us to see one another's face, smile at strangers, and connect with those around us. Not to mention the potential effects this could have on our children as they are told to stay home and go to school online, or go into school but to stay away from their classmates and wear a mask. It's devastating, but letting our children know why this is happening and that it won't last forever, along with encouraging them to have virtual hangouts with their friends, can help them get some of the connection they are missing. I have seen groups of parents getting tested for COVID-19, and once they receive the negative result, they form school groups or pods so that their children can engage socially and have some sort of normal school scenario. This pandemic has hit us hard, but we can adapt, lean on one another for support, and work to salvage some sense of normalcy during this trying time.

Social media allowed us to see what COVID-19 was doing to other parts of the world, first responders showing full hospitals, and people sharing videos of them and their loved ones waiting in long lines for treatment. The images, videos, and stories broke my heart and made it difficult for me to even get online for weeks at a time. The news stations had graphics with live tallies showing the number of cases and deaths thus far, and every story covered a new city being hit hard by this novel virus. I messaged my friends in Milan, Italy, to check in on them, only to hear that both of their parents had caught the virus. They were devastated and told me it felt as though they were living in a nightmare. They implored my husband and me to take it seriously, stay home, and wear our masks, because at this time they were about a month ahead of the US (based on when the first cases were recorded)—they felt that they could see into our future and they didn't want us to make the same mistakes. Luckily, both of their parents survived the virus and made full recoveries, but the impact of all that happened still lingers.

That was just the beginning: New York City (NYC) was one of the hardest-hit cities with over twenty-two thousand deaths.[7] It was eerie seeing the streets of NYC empty, and health-care workers showing red marks and bruises on their faces from wearing their personal protective equipment (PPE) as tightly as they could to ensure they were kept safe. To say we were overwhelmed during this time doesn't do it justice; I still remember watching the news as it showed large refrigerated trucks sitting outside of hospitals to help them manage all the bodies of those who had lost their lives to the virus. There were also companies in Brazil working to create cardboard hospital beds that also turn into coffins to help hospitals better manage the large number of deaths they were seeing every day.[8] The information online and on the news was unutterable. I felt so overcome with grief and sadness, and I wasn't even directly impacted. I cannot imagine the trauma felt by the people whose job it was to fill those refrigerated trucks, or treat those who were ill, not to mention all the people who still had to go into work during all of the chaos.

I have friends and family who were essential workers in grocery stores, prisons, and pharmacies. I felt compelled to call them every few days and check up on them, fearing that they would catch the virus and I wouldn't have gotten a chance to speak with them. The fear that we all felt for ourselves, our loved ones, and all who were affected was palpable and undeniable. We have never shared in trauma the way we have during the COVID-19 pandemic, and while it has been a complete tragedy, and many have lost their lives, it has also connected us, helped us to see that we are in this together, and brought out the best in people. One of my close friends has been checking on her elderly neighbors and going to the grocery store for them each week so they don't have to risk being infected, and many individuals have signed up for the vaccine trials, offering up their health to help others. In times like this, it can feel as though the good news is hard to find, but if we take the time to look for it, we will see that it's everywhere.

WHAT CAN WE DO TO SHAKE THIS TRAUMA EXPERIENCE?

We could talk about the COVID-19 pandemic for ages, there is so much still to process and learn, but what's important is figuring out how to deal with it. The reason this pandemic has been so harmful and upsetting isn't just because it's a virus, it's because we all felt threatened and therefore were pushed into our stress response. Our stress response is something that is only meant to be activated for a short period: we see a threat, we get ready to fight it or run from it, and we take action. For example, if we lived in a cave and heard a bear rustling the bushes outside, we would hear it, get scared, and run away. A few moments later, we would have reached a safe place, our stress response would no longer be necessary, and we would relax. However, when the threat we are all sensing is an invisible virus that we can catch from people and things, and we don't even know that much about it except that people are getting sick and dying, our body readies itself for fight, flight, or freeze. But there isn't any action we can take that will make the threat go away or be less scary. We have to sit in it, feeling the stress and energy course through our nervous system without a release.

The good news is that we can get that energy out and calm our nervous system down so that we feel better. The first tip and best way to do that is through true social connection. This is why COVID-19 hit us all so hard: We were threatened, stressed out, and then told to isolate to save lives. Doing the one thing we were told to do only made us feel worse, and that's why video calls became so popular and many people refused to follow the stay-at-home orders. We needed that connection to know that someone else understood us, and to be reminded that we are valued and important. Social connection has even been proven effective through Dr. Stephen Porges's polyvagal theory: instead of our nervous system being either more activated and less calm or calmer and less activated, it could do a little of both. We could be activated through social interaction while also calming our system down.[9] It's the safety we find in true connection with others that helps us manage and more quickly calm the stress response.

Another way to manage the stress or trauma we are experiencing is to take action where we can. Since our stress response readies our body for action, we have to move and do what we can to release it. We could start by cleaning the house or going for a walk, or what has helped me is dancing in my living room, which surprised me at first. Why did I feel so much better after dancing around for an hour to some music? Why did I feel worse on days when I didn't make time to dance? And then I remembered Dr. Peter Levine and somatic experiencing.

Dr. Levine studied animals in the wild and was interested in understanding why they could constantly be in traumatizing circumstances yet show no symptoms of trauma. What he found was that, after being in a threatening situation, animals either run or fight, then when they have gotten to a safer place, they do a full-body shake. They innately release all of their built-up energy so that they can relax. He believed that it was in our freeze state, when we aren't able to run or fight back, that trauma is born. This freeze experience can cause us to feel helpless, and immobilizes us, thus trapping the energy buildup in our body, leading to such symptoms of PTSD as hypervigilance, feeling on edge, dissociation, and flashbacks.[10] Making time to move our body can help regulate our nervous system and prevent any long-term symptoms of trauma—meaning that we can literally shake off some of the symptoms of trauma!

Also, it's best to limit the amount of media we digest each day. If we are only watching the number of cases and deaths go up, hearing interviews with people who have lost their jobs or someone they love, it's going to overwhelm us at one point or another. Not to mention that during times of stress and trauma, people are more irritable and easily angered, making social media a very toxic place to be. In the wake of COVID-19, I have seen more false facts, hate-filled comments, and passive-aggressive posts than ever before. I know we don't want to be ignorant of all that's happening in our world, but we don't have to engage with things 24/7 either, so find a balance that works for you. I decided to limit my news consumption to about thirty minutes each morning, and I only engage in social media when sharing my content or something positive I found. This allows me to stay informed yet not become overwhelmed with information, and it has drastically improved my mood.

Another way that we can manage the stress and trauma we feel is to consciously relax the muscles engaged during our stress response. These are the muscles in your face, neck, and shoulders. Keeping them tense will only perpetuate our body's trauma response and can even lead to muscle pain and headaches. Periodically throughout my day, I try to roll my shoulders down and back, do a few neck rolls in each direction, and relax my jaw. It sounds simple, but it works! When the pandemic first hit the US, I knew I was worried and stressed, but I didn't recognize that that was why my neck was killing me and I was constantly fighting tension headaches. Taking a few minutes each day to tense and then relax all of these muscles can help us notice when we are holding our emotional stress in our body and consciously let it go.

My final tip is to see a mental health professional. Having someone to vent to about all that we feel can not only lighten our emotional load, it can help us feel heard and valid in our thoughts and experience. This could also be the connection we are desperately needing right now, and the simple act of sharing space with another person could be calming in and of itself. We are all sharing in the trauma of the pandemic and talking about our experience with our therapist can deepen the therapeutic relationship and help us see them as people too. I cannot tell you the number of patients that have shared how comforting it is to know that I am struggling with this as well. In a way, the fact that I am upset, grieving, and stressed out validates their own experience and permits them to feel it too.

A few months into the COVID-19 pandemic, I released a video sharing how grief-stricken and upset I was with all that was going on in the world, and the reaction from my community was that of support and understanding. They, too, were sad, stressed out, and struggling to cope at home. I was nervous to release such a video because I don't usually share too much about myself or my struggles; I try to keep it educational and informative, but that didn't seem to work in this situation. No matter how many ways I tried to intellectualize, rationalize, and explain why I felt the way I felt, it didn't make me feel any better and it didn't lead to any helpful insights I could share with my community. I decided to just share my thoughts, unscripted and unedited, and it resonated more than I could have imagined. Hearing that I was sharing in their experience allowed them to accept how they were feeling, and instead of pretending that I knew better or had all the answers, I was now free to be in it with them. Sharing in trauma isn't pleasant, no one wants to be traumatized, but it sure is nice to not have to weather it alone.

I want you all to know that there is so much we can do to prevent the spread of trauma, from connecting with others to doing our work in therapy, to even just being more mindful of how we behave around our loved ones. Knowing that we can spread it is half the battle, and while chances are that we all will have at least one traumatic experience in our lifetime, that doesn't mean we have to let it change us or those around us. We can overcome it, we can get better, and we can heal. I think Dr. Peter Levine says it best: "Trauma is a fact of life; however, it doesn't have to be a life sentence."

KEY TAKEAWAYS

- Transgenerational trauma is trauma that is passed down from generation to generation—meaning that a child can express symptoms of PTSD without having been involved in any traumatic situation.

- Transgenerational trauma continues to be passed down for two main reasons: first, most of us don't realize we are struggling with it because we've never known another way; and second, healing from trauma is hard work.

- It's okay to talk to our children about how we are feeling, apologizing for times we got angry, and explaining why we are upset. However, we shouldn't expect any emotional support from our children; instead, we should seek out the help of a therapist or even a close friend.

- Trauma doesn't change our DNA, but it does change the epigenetic markers on our DNA. Epigenetic markers tell our brain and body how to read the DNA.

- Trauma can also be passed around to other people in our lives, not just those we are related to. Social media assists in this spread because it can give us more access to traumatizing situations.

- There are five ways we can manage our trauma response and stop the spread:

    1. Social connection. Making time to connect with loved ones can remind us we are not alone and help calm us down.
    2. Move our body! Shaking out the stress and fear helps regulate our system as well.
    3. Limit our exposure to the media. Not getting on social media or watching the news as often can help us curb our stress response.
    4. The muscles in our face, neck, and shoulders are involved in our stress response. Taking a minute to relax those muscles can help us feel better.
    5. Seeing a mental health professional. Having a safe space to vent and share all we may be feeling can not only give us the connection we may be craving but also validate our experience and get some helpful tips and tools along the way.

CHAPTER 9

WHY DO WE FEEL SO SCARED?

THE SCIENCE OF TRAUMA MEMORIES

H ave you ever been going about your day when you smell something familiar and it stops you in your tracks? Instantly, you are
reminded of another time, situation, or person; possibly you are
taken back for a moment to that time. It's as if that scent was somehow connected to a memory, and being around that smell pulls that
memory back to the surface. Just the other day, my husband and I
picked up some blueberries from the grocery store and when we got
them home and I popped one in my mouth, I was immediately taken
back to my childhood summers. When I was growing up, my cousin
Amanda and I would go to her grandparents' and swim in their pool
until our hair turned green, one of the side effects of being blond
and loving to swim. Outside of the fence surrounding the pool were
blueberry bushes, and we would run from the pool to the bushes
grabbing blueberries and quickly popping them into our mouth before going back to jump in the pool. The taste of a fresh blueberry
immediately takes me back to that time, and if I close my eyes I can
still smell the chlorine on my skin and hear the bees buzzing us as we
looked for ripe berries to pick. That was over twenty-five years ago,
yet through taste and smell, I can tap into that memory and feel as if
I am a kid again enjoying the warm summer sun.

Memories are interesting things. We count on them to help remind us where our car is parked, and also to recall that amazing
vacation we took, but we rarely give much thought to them. We can

take the creation and storage of memories for granted since it happens automatically. We go about our lives, and when asked about a certain time or situation, we can recall full details of an event or possibly just tidbits; either way, we can tap into our memory bank when needed. But how are memories formed? Why are some times and events easier to recall than others? Why do we sometimes have huge gaps in our memory? Are trauma memories different from regular ones? There is so much to learn, but we'll start with how they are created. Actually, let's try to make a memory together right now. I want you to think of these three terms: *palm tree, flip-flop,* and *water bottle.* Try to put these three terms into a story, and maybe even spray your favorite scent into the air or onto this book. Smell that scent, think of those terms, and I will check in later to see whether you can remember them.

HOW ARE MEMORIES CREATED?

The hippocampus is the part of the temporal lobe in our brain that's responsible for memory creation as well as for storing long-term memory. Researchers have also looked at the brains of people who had Alzheimer's disease and discovered a profound loss of cells in the hippocampus, while other areas remained intact[1]—thus proving that our hippocampus is the area of the brain responsible for memory function and retention.

How the hippocampus stores our memories, or whether they are kept there, is up for debate, but we do know that memories themselves come from patterns of neuronal activity that can be ignited through our environment—meaning that when I taste that fresh blueberry, the set of neurons associated with that memory are activated and connect to mentally take me back to that time I enjoyed them poolside as a child. These neurons are like a group of old friends getting back together to help us recall that information. As we grow and develop, our hippocampus creates more of these neurons through a process called neurogenesis, and each day they join together to form new memories. That's why when we smell or taste something, for example, we can be pulled back into a memory. The smell or taste triggered those neurons associated with that memory to get back together and play it back for us. But if we don't access those neurons very often, they can forget about one another or what to do when triggered, and our brain will eventually clean out the ones not being used, to make space for the newer or stronger memories.[2]

One of my favorite representations of memory creation and storage is shown in the Disney Pixar movie *Inside Out*. As the viewer, you get to see inside the mind of a young girl named Riley and watch as her emotions control what she thinks and does. They manage her memory recall and even send her newly formed memories from that day to long-term memory when she goes to sleep. I love this film because the way her emotions—which are depicted as characters— show memory creation and management is surprisingly accurate. Each memory is represented as a perfectly formed marble, and they share how Riley's core memories power the different pillars of her personality. They also accurately show how memories can change after they have been formed, because our perspective has shifted or we have been through a different experience. Since our memories are formed through connections in neurons, we can add to an older memory when we come into contact with new information—meaning we just added some newer neurons to an older neuron bundle.

Something I have noticed over my years of creating video content online is that I am not able to tell the same story twice. That doesn't mean that I can't get the same points across, or remember the key components to it, but it won't ever be exactly the same. Every time I share a memory or explanation about something, it's unique, and the precise wording can't be re-created. How we tell a story about our life can be impacted by how we feel that day, how well rested we are, or what point we are trying to make. Every time we reach into our memory bank to tell a story, that memory returns with a few changes. In *Inside Out*, Riley's emotions pull up one of her old happy memories, but the character Sadness touches the memory while it's playing and alters it. Another character, Joy, attempts to change it back but can't, and tells Sadness to not touch any more memories until they can figure out how to fix what she did.

The truth is, we can't change them back. We now have new information and have applied that to what we knew, and in a way, it's helpful, adaptive, and allows us to be educated and grow. It's also important to know that memories cannot be changed unless they are brought into our conscious mind; it's only in the retrieval and reliving of them that we can change them. So, it's easy to conclude that if we haven't recalled something until now, there is no way we could have made it up, or altered it, which will be important to remember as we discuss trauma memories.[3]

HOW ARE MEMORIES STORED?

One important component of memory creation and storage is sleep. In *Inside Out*, Riley's emotions wait until she goes into REM (rapid eye movement) sleep before hitting the button to move all her newly created memories to be filed away in her long-term memory bank. What occurs during our REM sleep is that our hippocampus repeatedly reactivates the newly encoded materials—meaning that it takes newly formed memories and triggers the neurons over and over so that we can form a strong memory that can be easily recalled at a later time. This process, called memory consolidation, is imperative for learning and memory formation. That's why sleep researchers, such as Dr. Matthew Walker, talk endlessly about the importance of sleep: though each of us will have different needs, we all require at least seven and a half hours of sleep a night to ensure our brain and body function well the following day. If we don't get enough sleep, it can cause a buildup of newly formed memories without strong connections to clog up our hippocampus and make it harder for us to learn new things or recall things we learned before.[4]

Dr. Walker said something interesting when he was on Joe Rogan's podcast. He stated that when we are sleeping in a hotel or away from home, we don't get the same quality of sleep because only half of our brain can sleep, leaving the other half to stay up and be on guard. It's a sort of protective mechanism within our system to ensure that when we are in a new location, we are kept safe.[5] If we apply this to trauma, knowing that those who struggle with C-PTSD may have never felt safe, or gotten a full night's sleep, always feeling on edge or threatened, it's no wonder many struggle with their memories of that time. Their hippocampus never had the chance to consolidate what happened to form an easily retrievable memory.

ARE TRAUMA MEMORIES DIFFERENT?

If our memories are like the marbles shown in *Inside Out*, then a trauma memory would be a shattered marble, dropped on the floor of our hippocampus; it wasn't fully formed and it couldn't be consolidated and sent off to long-term memory. The splinters are everywhere, and when we least expect it, we can step on one and be pulled back into a fraction of that trauma memory. I have heard from many of my patients that these trauma memories can be difficult to untangle, and the longer we go without processing them, the more confusing they become. Many talk about them as being like hazy dreams that don't make any sense, or like an image that's so out of focus that they can't tell what it is.

Another reason that trauma memories can be so confusing is that the sheer act of remembering them triggers our stress response, activating our amygdala. When our amygdala is activated, it overrides our prefrontal cortex, which is the control center in our brain. Its job is to help us plan, put feelings into words, consider the options we have available, and make the decision that's best for us. In many ways, our prefrontal cortex is responsible for our personality, and what makes us who we are. If it's offline, we can't think clearly—we can only think of how to get out of this threatening situation, and we use our emotional response to aid us in our escape. I believe this is why, for many of us, trauma memories are just too stressful or emotional to recall, and why we can't see it clearly or remember the details; all we can do is remember the feeling.

That's why it's no surprise to find out that the amygdala is connected to the hippocampus—meaning that our emotion and threat response is linked to the part of the brain responsible for memory. Which makes sense, because our memories of events do have emotions attached to them. As I recall those summers at the pool with my cousin, I feel joyful, relaxed, and maybe a little sad that we don't have summers like that anymore. So much of our memories are tied up in our emotions, and if one is too upsetting or emotionally driven, it can trigger our stress response, stimulating our amygdala.

If the amygdala is activated, and other areas are turned off, it could be igniting our emotions about a situation without any context, and why we only remember how we felt, not what happened to us. Psychiatrists and neuroscientists believe that because the role of the amygdala is to recognize a threat and ready us to deal with

> As I have attempted to talk through these memories with my therapist, all I can remember is how I felt. I have flashes of feeling scared, trapped, and helpless. But I can't come up with any of the details about what happened, just what it felt like, and sometimes I can't even come up with that. It's like once I start to remember bits of what happened to me I dissociate, and come to in my car on my way home from my therapy session. And that's terrifying too!

it, it's constantly using our senses to check out our environment. This can help prevent us from getting into threatening situations, and allow us to more quickly recognize something dangerous, but it can also lead to us associating benign items with the harmful event. For example, if I were sexually abused by a neighbor, and this abuse occurred after they gave me a snack of crackers and peanut butter, I might connect that snack, or even just the smell of those items, with the abuse. If I find myself at a friend's house years later, and they use that same brand of peanut butter, I can be triggered by the smell or taste of it. Even if I don't remember what happened to me, my brain knows that when I smell or taste things like that, I am hurt, and it readies me for action.[6]

These sensory connections can continue to grow and spread as we have other traumatizing situations or remember other bits of what's happened to us—making it even more difficult for us to know what occurred and manage all of the triggers we encounter every day. It's as if the cards are stacked against us when we are traumatized. We can't sleep well because of the nightmares or just not being safe in our own home, therefore our brain cannot fully process or consolidate the memory. This means that we can't fully remember what happened, other than the emotions we felt or just flashes of the experience. Finally, our amygdala continues to add more and more triggers to the list to try to keep us safe, but instead, it can make almost any object or person a reminder of the terrifying event. In many cases, this can leave us feeling frozen with fear for much of our life, struggling to have relationships and function in daily activities.

DID I MAKE IT UP?

When every bit you know about an upsetting event seems to flash in and out of focus, not make sense, and change all the time, it can be hard to know whether we are making it all up. Too often, I hear from

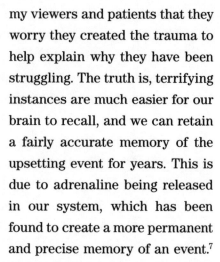

> My memories feel like they have gone through many 'sieves,' ones with big holes and ones with tiny holes, to the point where I don't even know what really happened, what has been told to me, or what I could have made up.

my viewers and patients that they worry they created the trauma to help explain why they have been struggling. The truth is, terrifying instances are much easier for our brain to recall, and we can retain a fairly accurate memory of the upsetting event for years. This is due to adrenaline being released in our system, which has been found to create a more permanent and precise memory of an event.[7]

Also, we already know that memories cannot be altered without their being remembered, so it's very unlikely that we made up a traumatic instance.

This may seem off base, but I love the show *Law & Order*, and every time the characters go out to ask the neighbors or other people on the street whether they saw anything odd or heard anything strange that day, for the most part, these individuals don't recall hearing or seeing anything. That's because, if they hadn't encountered something scary or unsettling, no adrenaline would have pumped through their system to help form an accurate and long-lasting memory. If we experience only things that seem normal and regular, we don't remember them as well. For example, we may all clearly remember where we were on 9/11, but it's not as likely that we will remember what we were doing the day or week before.

Although adrenaline can help us form more clear and lasting memories, it helps us only up to a certain point. If we, as Bessel van der Kolk states in his book *The Body Keeps the Score*, "are confronted with horror—especially the horror of 'inescapable shock'—this system becomes overwhelmed and breaks down."[8] This is what leads to these fragments of memory and bits of emotional and sensory reminders without any story to make sense of them. In a way, we know what happened, while at the same time, we don't.

Since trauma memories can have many environmental triggers, we will constantly be pulled back into pieces of the memory and experience bits of it over and over until we process it. I have always thought that this occurrence, while extremely uncomfortable, is a good sign. Our brain doesn't often allow us to recall any trauma memory while we are still in a dangerous situation. It hides the memory away so that we can live through the traumatic situation and be okay. It's like it sweeps the splinters of that shattered marble under the rug until we are safe and then pulls the rug away to remind us of what's there when we have made it to safety. Therefore, flashbacks and bits of memory returning to the surface mean that we are doing okay, and now is the time to process all that happened.

Memories of my childhood trauma used to be kind of a huge, blurry, yet familiar memory, kind of like when you wake up and half recall a dream. While I was being treated for trauma at the VA, individual memories would come into focus. As soon as they came into focus, there would be a relief of finally resolving that blurry memory, like when you have a word on the tip of your tongue and then realize what the word is.

Trauma memories aren't like other memories. We are not in control of when we recall them, and they don't fade away as normal memories do either. We can go about our lives for years thinking nothing has happened, only to run into an environmental trigger and suddenly realize that something terrible occurred.

Normal or nontraumatizing memories aren't like that; there's never a period when we aren't able to remember what it was like to graduate from college, or what happened on our wedding day.

Normal memories aren't completely forgotten only to resurface later; that's only something trauma memories do. If someone was to ask you about one of the happiest days of your life, you would probably think for a bit, get a smile on your face, and recall a beginning, middle, and end to your story. You could easily come up with the story of that day, and it would make sense. Trauma memories, on the other hand, are disorganized, unclear, and don't follow any timeline. We can mix up what happened to us when we were seven with another event that occurred when we were twelve. All of those splinters are mixed together, and since we didn't get an opportunity to piece them together and file it away, we can't easily remember what happened when.

CAN WE TRUST TRAUMA MEMORIES?

Because trauma memories are disorganized, fleeting, and difficult to recall, many victims of trauma worry that they are making up their memories. Going our whole life without thinking we were hurt, only to come into contact with something and have a terrifying memory come flooding back is odd. We can think there's no way it's true, we must be going crazy! Not to mention that we may not get the entire memory back at once; we may only get a feeling or a flash of ourselves in a hurtful position, and it's tough to make sense of that.

A few years ago, I had a patient who had come to me for help with his depressive symptoms. It had caused him to gain weight and lose his girlfriend of two years, and he was currently struggling to keep up with college classes. It was due to the urging of his parents that he reached out for my help. For months, we worked together to combat negative and motivation-stealing thoughts, and slowly things began to improve. About six months into our work together, his family took a trip back East to visit some extended family they hadn't seen in years. My patient was a bit nervous; he hadn't seen these members of his family since he was a child, and he also hadn't missed his weekly session with me since we began. We went over the tools that had worked for him so far, prepared him for the trip, and planned for a phone session. I remember thinking that this trip was going to be good for him because he would get to test out some of his new skills in a safe space with a family that cared about him. I thought it would help him build some much-needed self-confidence, and I was excited to hear how it was going in our phone session.

A few days into his trip, I received a panicked voicemail asking me to please call him back immediately; he was not doing well and needed help. I was shocked, and when I returned his call, he frantically told me about how they all went out for dinner the other night, and when he gave his uncle a hug, he suddenly remembered something. He couldn't piece it together at first, but he said he knew something bad had happened to him at the hands of his uncle. He said the smell of his cologne brought up these memories of being in his swimsuit in a damp basement and being scared. He saw flashes of himself naked in this light yellow bathroom, being washed by someone. He told me he felt sick to his stomach and spent the entire dinner "totally spaced out," not sure what was going on. Unfortunately, coming into contact with his abuser after all these years uncovered a deeply hidden trauma memory, and because of the intense shock of this revelation, he dissociated. I kept in daily contact with him while he was on vacation, and told him to stay away from his uncle as much as possible. It was a rough week, but he made it back and we started working to help him heal from this past trauma.

While some people may balk at the idea of repressed memories (otherwise known as dissociative amnesia), wondering how someone could forget something so terrible, remember that this is part of the diagnostic criteria for PTSD: "inability to remember an important aspect of the traumatic event(s) (typically due to dissociative amnesia and not to other factors such as head injury, alcohol, or drug(s)."[9] There has been a research battle going on for years about whether repressed memories are real, but if I'm honest, I don't care about being right or following the research as much as I care about helping my patients and viewers feel heard and understood.

One of the biggest arguments against the existence of repressed memories is that there isn't any evidence to support that the repression occurs without conscious effort—meaning that these trauma memories don't just hide away on their own; we choose to conceal them ourselves.[10] I don't know about you, but I don't think that proves anything. How the forgetting began isn't as important as whether people fully forget what occurred, and we have plenty of research to support that it does.

One important study about repressed memories that van der Kolk references is "Recall of Childhood Trauma: A Prospective Study of Women's Memories of Child Sexual Abuse," conducted by Dr. Linda Meyer Williams in the early 1970s and published in 1994. Williams completed sit-down interviews with 206 girls immediately following their admission into the hospital for sexual abuse, and all of the victims spoke about the abuse they had just endured. Then, seventeen years later, she reinterviewed 136 of the original 206 girls and found that 12 percent of them said they were never abused in their lifetime, 38 percent

> These memories are so hard to recall because I don't really want to remember; it's like my brain holds its hands up and goes, 'No that's too much, I can't handle that.' So, it's buried deep until you feel safe enough to process whatever it is. I also think recall is hard because of shame. For me, I feel ashamed that I ever let bad things happen in the first place, remembering them would be a difficult experience. I also worry I've made experiences up, because I can't fully recall it due to how painful it is, or I feel like I let it happen because things like that don't happen to people.

did not remember the abuse she had recorded years earlier, and 68 percent of them reported new incidents of childhood sexual abuse not already in their files.

Williams also looked into the reliability of the girls' memories and found that the younger the victims were when the abuse occurred, the more likely they were to forget it at some point in their lives. In fact, 16 percent of those who did recall their abuse said that they had forgotten about it at some point in the last seventeen years but then remembered it again later on. Also, the victims who remembered the abuse when reinterviewed by Williams were able to recall much of what they told her all those years ago. Some of the minor details had changed, but the core facts and story of the trauma stayed the same. This proves that even if we do forget about our trauma for a period, we can still accurately recall the events, and therefore we can trust our trauma memories.

As I have talked through memories, I realized that my brain has tried to completely detach myself from what happened, which has led to me questioning myself and whether these events really happened. Whenever I talk or write about these memories, it feels like I am talking about someone else. It's like my mind can't come to terms with the fact that this happened to me and is something very real that I need to work through.

I know that some memories are too difficult to manage at the time; therefore, we return to them when we can finally process them through. I also believe that just because our brain doesn't repress the memories without us consciously making them, that doesn't make the memories themselves any less real or true. In many ways, our brain and body are adaptive, and we hide things away until we feel safe to pull them back out again; it's something we feel we must do to survive. When we are still being traumatized, or are unsafe, we are not going to have the energy or motivation that's required to process an upset like that. All of our drive must support our survival and escape from the terrorizing situation.

WHAT IF OUR MEMORIES AREN'T COMPLETE?

For most of my patients, the trauma memories don't just come flooding back with all the details and particulars we have been looking for. Instead, they trickle in slowly, revealing more and more information as we seek it out. This process can be difficult, slow, and confusing at times, because not all of the memories that come back are actual trauma memories. Remember what we talked about previously? That our amygdala can associate trauma and upset with all sorts of different objects, making our ability to recall the core instance all the more difficult? It can cause our recollection of an event to be tied up with a ton of triggers and flashes of fear that shouldn't be linked to the terrorizing event itself. We can struggle to know what happened when, and what triggers are real. One way to make sense of all this splintered information is to create a trauma timeline, which is exactly what it sounds like—a drawn or written-out chronological account of what has happened in our life. We want to identify the main upsetting events and place them on the timeline with as much accuracy as we can. One important thing to remember when organizing our memories is to not get too caught up in whether something is a trauma. Big-T and little-T traumas all have a place on this timeline, as well as times when we felt calm or happy.

Keeping a timeline as a living document allows us to fill it in as more memories come flooding back. It can help us see all we have been through and validate why we may be having a tough time, as well as help us recognize patterns of behavior in our families. Many of my patients have said that seeing it all written out stops it from getting more confusing or their feeling that they have to keep it all straight in their head. Breaking down our lifetime into five-year increments is a good place to start, and fill in each chunk with whatever comes to mind when you think of that period. These could be things like our parent's divorce, moving, changing schools, abuse, addiction in our home, first sexual experience, fighting with a friend, and so on.

Doing the work of putting together a trauma timeline helps us place our upsetting memories into narrative form, which can be healing too. It's often the lack of verbal or storied memory that keeps us from processing what happened and filing it away in our long-term memory and can cause us to continue struggling with flashbacks and other symptoms of PTSD. Therefore, putting words to what happened, keeping it in a cohesive timeline, and being validated along the way can help us make some sense of what happened. For many years, most mental health professionals, myself included, believed that talking through trauma would help our patients heal and move on. However, upon further research and experience, we know that though talk therapy does help some people heal, most of us with PTSD will need additional forms of treatment to achieve full remission of our symptoms.

Talking through what happened in a cohesive story is a good place to start on our path to recovery, but for many of us, even this first step feels impossible. What if we still have periods where we don't remember anything? How can we check to make sure we are putting the pieces together properly? How can we fact-check this? One of the most helpful tools in this portion of trauma work is to find a fact-checker. A fact-checker is someone in your life that you feel comfortable talking to, who would know whether something you remember is true. They can fill in any blanks you may still have and offer up other tidbits of information to help you make sense of the rest of your timeline or story.

It can be hard to find someone like this, but the first place to look is to a sibling, preferably an older one. If we don't have a sibling,

> When I remember a memory now it feels as if it happened to someone else. I can recall what has happened but not the emotions with it, or the opposite way around. Sometimes it still makes me believe that it's all in my head until I talk to someone older that has remembered what happened to reassure my thoughts.

or we don't get along with the ones we do have, we can look to a cousin, aunt, or even a babysitter—anyone who would have been around during that time who could help us piece things together. Now, I know this can be scary; we are opening up to someone regarding things that we still aren't sure about, and they could tell us what we remember didn't happen. They could retraumatize us or cause us to feel we are back at square one. That's why we don't reach out to other people until we have worked on the timeline and story for a while, when we have some specific questions for them. We don't ask our fact-checkers whether something happened, we tell them what we remember, and ask direct questions, such as, "Hey, remember when we used to camp by the lake every summer? I remember this one year when we had fireworks, and one shot right at me—was it our uncle who set those off, or someone else?" We let them know what we remember and ask them for one or two clarifying things. This keeps it on topic and prevents them from potentially adding details that aren't helpful to us and our healing.

Taking the time to untangle our memories and piece together what happened to us can be difficult, overwhelming, and at times unbearable. For those reasons, we must give ourselves the time and space needed to do the work. So often, I hear how much people wish they could speed things up, heal more quickly, and just get over it already. The secret to consolidating and healing from these trauma memories is in the letting go of the result and allowing ourselves to go at the pace we can. Too often, in recovery, we want to push harder, move faster, and force our brain into submission, but that can end up doing more harm than good. Instead of expecting our process to follow a certain schedule, we should try to accept where we are at, let go of the things we cannot change, and allow ourselves the time needed to heal. Some things in life cannot be rushed, and trauma work is one of those, so be compassionate with yourself as you move through it, and trust me, it does get better.

KEY TAKEAWAYS

- Memories are created in our hippocampus, which connects groups of neurons to one another. They are saved in this long-term memory bank during our REM sleep cycle.

- The sheer act of retrieving an older memory changes it slightly because we have new experiences and perspectives to add to it.

- Trauma memories are different because they aren't complete and therefore cannot be logged away into our long-term memory. By trying to remember them, we trigger our amygdala, which can make putting our feelings to words even more difficult and prevent us from making sense of what happened.

- Our amygdala continues to add an increasing number of triggers to the list to try to keep us safe, but instead, it can make almost any object or person a reminder of the terrifying event. This can make trauma memories confusing and hard to understand.

- Trauma memories are not like regular memories, because we don't control when they are recalled, nor do they fade away as normal memories do.

- Repressed memories are real; however, we do consciously push them down. Once we retrieve them, they are found to be accurate and trustworthy.

- If there are gaps in our memory due to trauma, using a trauma timeline, putting our experiences into a narrative, and finding fact-checkers from that time can help us figure out what happened.

- Trauma memories take time to put together, so be patient with ourselves and our process, because it does get better.

CHAPTER 10

HOW CAN WE RECOVER?

THE BENEFITS OF NEUROPLASTICITY

W e have all heard the adage that you can't teach an old dog new tricks. We tend to use this phrase when we encounter someone who is stubborn in their ways or isn't open to any feedback about the way they handle things. We often let older people off the hook with this proverb, believing that it's better to just let them be the way they are, and not bother them with any expectation of change. However, the truth is that everyone, no matter their age, learns new things every day through a process called neuroplasticity. The term *neuroplasticity* was introduced in 1906 by Italian psychiatrist Ernesto Lugaro, and it explains why we can adapt, learn, and grow throughout our lives[1]—meaning that no matter how old we get, we can be taught new tricks!

Neuroplasticity allows for our nervous system to be shaped or molded; in other words, with enough energy and repetition, we can change our brain. This is where the field of psychology thrives; this career is founded in the belief that people can change, heal, and grow, and it's up to us mental health professionals to guide them on their way. We discussed in the last chapter how our brain creates new neurons every day, and it's with those neurons that it builds new memories; we also learned that it gets rid of the unused information to make room for all of these new skills and experiences. It's in this daily churn that we learn new things and make room for change.

HOW CAN I LEARN NEW TRICKS?

When I was a kid, I used to bite my nails, and even though I hated that I did it, I couldn't stop. My mom thought it was a bad habit that would lead to my getting sick more often because my fingers were constantly in my mouth, and so she tried to help. She bought this bad-tasting nail polish, offered me rewards for not biting my nails, yet nothing seemed to work until I told my friend Helen about it. She swore that she would get me to stop, and began batting my hand away any time I tried to bite my nails. She would even shout at me to stop when I was out of arm's reach. At first, it was funny, and I would sometimes still bite my nails (often to be stubborn or show her that I couldn't be stopped), but her consistent hitting and shouting made me more aware of when I was biting my nails, and after a while, the behavior ceased. Every time I would raise my hand to my mouth, I could hear her screaming for me to stop, or feel an arm reaching out to swat my hand away. This consistent punishment, while play-ful, slowly decreased my urge to bite my nails, and I haven't done it since.

I know that talking about how I stopped biting my nails when we are discussing trauma can seem like an oversight or insensitive, but I think it's important we understand how we learn in basic situations before applying it to bigger issues like traumatic events. Let's start by getting into the three types of behavioral learning: classical con-ditioning, operant conditioning, and observational learning.

Classical conditioning had the most influence on this area of psy-chology, and to share one of my favorite psychology jokes of all time, does the name Pavlov ring a bell? If you don't get that joke now, don't worry, it will all make sense soon. Classical conditioning is when we pair a neutral stimulus with a naturally occurring response. This type of conditioning was accidentally discovered in a famous study conducted by Russian physiologist Ivan Pavlov in the 1890s. Pavlov originally believed that dogs would salivate when food was placed in front of them, which makes sense. If they see and smell the food, of course, they would salivate; it's how our digestive system begins its process. However, what he found was that the dogs would begin salivating when they would hear the footsteps of his assistants who were getting the food ready. They had learned that the sound of their footsteps meant food was coming, and their body readied itself for it. Upon seeing this behavior, he wanted to test this discovery and hypothesis: that you could pair a neutral stimulus with a naturally occurring response.

Pavlov reconstructed his study to include a bell being rung before the food was given to the dogs. He wanted to see whether he could pair this neutral stimulus (the sound of a bell) to the dogs' natural response when they saw food (salivation). Each time the assistants fed the dogs, they would ring the bell first, and then place their food in front of the animals. Slowly, the dogs began to associate the sound of the bell with being fed, and then by just ringing the bell, Pavlov could cause the dogs to salivate. This was the first proof that classical conditioning worked, and Pavlov devoted the rest of his career to studying it.[2] Now, do you understand my joke? It's just so dorky and funny, and feel free to use it at your next party.

What this style of learning means for us is that, if we have a trigger or stimulus in our life that is causing us pain or upset, we can in fact pair that stimulus with something more positive and, in essence, snuff out the negative connection. A current example of this would be the fact that social gatherings have resulted in an increase in COVID-19 cases and deaths. Therefore, we can begin to associate getting together with others with sickness and death, and feel the urge to isolate completely. However, once we have a vaccine and treatment, we can slowly expose ourselves to others in a safe and healthy way, and will be able to see that fewer people get sick, and more are able to recover. By slowly exposing ourselves to the scary thing (gathering) without getting the terrifying result, we can change our previous association. This is not only exciting to know, but it also offers hope for a better future for those of us who have felt imprisoned by our past experiences.

The next type of behavioral learning is the one we hear about and use the most, and it's called operant conditioning. Operant conditioning is what I described with my friend Helen and my desire to stop biting my nails; through her consistent punishment when I tried to bite my nails, I was able to decrease that behavior. The most famous study related to operant conditioning was conducted by B. F. Skinner in the 1930s and used what he called the "Skinner box" to demonstrate how reinforcement and punishment can shape behavior. Skinner would place hungry rats into this box that had a lever on the side of it. When the rats began running around the box, they would inadvertently hit the lever and a food pellet would come out. It didn't take very long for the rats to learn that when they were hungry, they just hit that lever and food would come out. The food was known as a positive reinforcement since it reinforced the behavior that the rats' hitting the lever yielded food and made it more likely that they would hit that lever over and over again.

Another way to strengthen certain behavior is by removing an adverse stimulus, otherwise known as negative reinforcement. In the Skinner box, this form of reinforcement was demonstrated by electrifying the floor of the box, making the rats uncomfortable and causing them to run quickly around the box. They would accidentally bump into the lever, causing the electricity to stop, and their discomfort would go away. It didn't take long before they learned that the lever would stop the shock, and when the rats were placed back into the Skinner box, they would quickly make their way over to the lever and hit it. They had learned through negative reinforcement to hit that lever and to do it quickly.[3]

When I was in college we had this computer game called "Sniffy the Virtual Rat" that allowed us to conduct studies just like B. F. Skinner, but without harming any rats, and it was interesting to see how such a simple positive or negative reinforcement could change their behavior. I also enjoyed the fact that through technological advancements, we could get away from having to use real animals in our studies, because I don't know whether I could have completed my homework using a real rat, especially as we got into the punishment portion of the study.

While positive and negative reinforcements seemed to shape the behavior of the rats, Skinner also tried punishment as a means of weakening or removing the reinforced behavior—meaning that when the rat would get into the box and begin hitting the lever, it would get a small electrical shock. This was done to see how quickly this punishment could extinguish the already learned behavior (to hit the lever), and though this did work, and the rats quickly stopped hitting the lever, it also made them fear the lever. Some became aggressive, and it didn't guide them toward any desired behavior, only away from the undesired one. Overall, what this tells us is that if we want to change our behavior or the behavior of our children, it's best if we use positive or negative reinforcement. Having a reward added or a negative situation removed allows us to shape our behavior into something more positive and helpful while avoiding any unfavorable side effects.

The final type of behavioral learning is observational learning, which is when we master something by watching someone else do it and imitating their behavior. This happens a lot in children, and we have that funny saying "Monkey see, monkey do," which represents the art of mimicking or imitating. If we watch someone do something enough times, we can usually figure out how to do it ourselves.

When I was growing up, we had a lot of animals—multiple dogs, cats, and guinea pigs—and they would all watch us open up the doors in the house or the ones in their cages every day. Since our yard was not fully fenced, we would put our dogs into the kennel before leaving for an outing, and one summer I remember walking out to lock them in, and when I got back inside my mom asked why I hadn't put the dogs away yet. I was stumped, because I had just put them in the kennel. She went out and placed them in herself and we left for the afternoon, and when we returned, the dogs were back out in the yard. We figured they had gotten out somehow, but couldn't figure it out because it looked as if their kennel door was still closed. We put them back in the kennel and then looked through the window in the house to see our golden retriever Bailey carefully balance on his back legs while lifting the latch, opening the door, and then shutting it behind him. We were shocked and amazed, and immediately got a different latch that didn't just hook over the pole on their kennel, and they never got out again.

I would like to say this was the only case of our animals learning from observing us, but our cats also figured out how to open the pantry door so that they could get into their food, and our guinea pigs found a way to let themselves out of their cage. Observational learning is probably our most innate form of learning and part of why studying in school with others is so beneficial. This is also why many parents try their best to model good behavior for their children; they are watching us and picking up on our actions and language. One of my favorite observational learning stories comes from my babysitting days in college. I used to babysit for this couple who had just had twins, and the mom would have me pop by for a few hours so that she could get things done around the house, visit friends, or go run errands. One day, it was my duty to get the twins to their Gymboree class, and so I strapped them into their car seats, packed up their snacks, and we hopped onto the freeway. If you don't live in a city like Los Angeles, know that you rarely just hop on the freeway; it's more of a battle, and traffic seems to happen no matter what day or time you are traveling. This day was no different, and as we came to a stop on the on-ramp, one of the twins let out a big sigh and said, "Well, shit, traffic again," as she threw her arms at her side and dropped her head. I burst out laughing but quickly pulled myself together so that I didn't reinforce her behavior. When I got back to the house, I let her mom know what had happened, and she admitted that she wasn't the best at watching what she said when the twins were in the car, and we both had a good laugh about it.

The goal is to understand that there are many ways in which we can change and grow, and I believe this can easily be applied to therapy and healing from past trauma. For example, observational learning can happen in therapy, as a therapist demonstrates healthy communication, understanding, and even how to disagree without aggression. We can also incorporate some positive reinforcement in therapy or even do it ourselves in our own life. I have even done this with my book-writing process. Each week, I have some small goals I hope to accomplish, whether that's how much research I hope to complete or a certain number of pages I want to finish. If I reach those goals, then I reward myself at the end of the week. It keeps me motivated and makes it easier for me to jump back into writing in the following weeks and months. In therapy, I can apply this in the same way, working with a patient to come up with some small goals, such as trying to expose themselves to a triggering item and using their new tools to calm themselves back down. If they do this successfully once this week, they will have a reward already planned, such as getting a coffee, taking a week off from therapy homework, or buying themselves something.

HOW DO I CHANGE MY BEHAVIOR?

When it comes to behavioral change in trauma work, we must go beyond the learning models and dig into our thoughts because, like it or not, thoughts are the drivers of our actions, and of how we can make real, lasting change in our brain and life. One of the best styles of therapy for this is cognitive behavioral therapy (CBT), since it works under the belief that our thoughts lead to our feelings, which, in turn, lead to our behaviors. This creates a sort of cycle as we go through life—while we are engaging in certain behaviors, they can work to only intensify our original thoughts, and there we are back at the beginning of that cycle again.

Since I know this can be hard to visualize, let me share a personal example. For years, I have struggled with overapologizing, even saying sorry for saying "Sorry" too much; I know, it was bad. But this issue all stemmed from my thoughts about my existence. I would often have thoughts like "I am not good enough" or "I am just not getting the hang of this fast enough, I am letting people down," and because of those thoughts, I would feel sad, lesser than, and that I just wanted to disappear. All of those thoughts and feelings would lead me to overapologize. I would assume that my boss didn't think I was catching on quickly enough and so I'd apologize for how long it took me to complete a task, or I would worry that I was in someone's way in the grocery store and say sorry as I moved my cart to another part of the aisle. As I engaged in these behaviors, I was only solidifying my thoughts and feelings that I was less than and not good enough. It had been pointed out to me throughout my life: once my softball coach told me that I would have to run the bases every time I said sorry to him when it wasn't warranted, and I ran almost the entire practice. But it wasn't until my husband, Sean, started to kindly point it out that I brought it up in therapy and decided I needed to change.

Just like any change we want to make, it took time and a lot of work. My therapist had me start noticing what my thoughts were in situations where I felt the urge to apologize; in CBT, this is called keeping a thought record. She had me write down some of these thoughts, and surprisingly, a lot of them were just different versions of the same thoughts. I was having these repetitive negative thoughts about myself all day every day. Which kind of sucked to realize, but was also validating in that I had proof that my urge to constantly apologize was coming from somewhere. She had me continue to keep track of my thoughts while also journaling about how I felt and what I did each day.

Next, my therapist discussed cognitive distortions with me, which is just a fancy phrase for thoughts or beliefs we have that are not founded in any truth. There are ten main cognitive distortions: all-or-nothing thinking, overgeneralizations, discounting positive things that happen, filtering, jumping to conclusions, emotional reasoning, magnification, labeling, "should" statements, and self-blame.[4] My biggest distortion was "should" statements. I believed that I should be better, faster, smarter, or whatever, and therefore I needed to apologize constantly to make up for the fact that I could never meet my unattainable goals or standards. In a way, I was setting myself up for failure.

WHAT DO MY THOUGHTS HAVE TO DO WITH IT?

Before we move on to the next step in my CBT work, I want to explain each of the cognitive distortions or faulty thoughts because we all have them, and we must understand them so we are able to more quickly identify them in our life. First up is all-or-nothing thinking, or what I like to call the diet mentality: I am either on a diet, eating perfectly, or I am not on a diet, so I might as well eat everything in sight. We could also call this distortion black-or-white thinking, because it doesn't leave room for any slipups, mistakes, or possibility of it getting better. It only sees things as one way or another, all or nothing.

Next, we have overgeneralizations, and this happens when we take one experience and apply that result to everything else in our lives. We can assume, because we had one bad relationship where someone hurt us, that all relationships we could be in will end the same way. Generalizing like this doesn't leave any room for change and loves such words as "always" and "never."

Moving on, discounting positive things that happen is a very common cognitive distortion in my patients with anxiety or depression.

We can have a pretty wonderful day, everything is going our way, people are kind, and we accomplish what we need to; however, when we get home, we get into an argument with our daughter, and then we think our entire day, hell, our entire life, is shit. We can overlook any of the good things that have taken place and instead focus on the one bad thing. This doesn't allow us to see the full picture or manage life's ups and downs.

Filtering is the combination of overgeneralizing and negating the positive. This happens when we only focus on one bad part of an experience, magnify all of the details, and obsess over it so that we can't see any of the positive things about it or ourselves. It filters out all of the other information or facts so that we only see what we want to see.

There is also the cognitive distortion of jumping to conclusions, which I think we all do from time to time. We can do this by assuming we can read someone's mind, that we know they are upset, angry, or hate us. Because of this thought distortion, we can act in ways that support those thoughts and harm our relationships. We can also do this by thinking we can see into the future and act a certain way because we "know what's going to happen." Again, this doesn't allow for life to unfold or thoughts to be challenged, because we are taking action that only solidifies the false thoughts.

Another cognitive distortion that I see constantly in my office and online is emotional reasoning, where we judge ourselves or our environment based on how we feel. For example, if we are having a bad day and feeling stressed out, we can believe that that one person on the Zoom call not muting their mic while they do things around the house is doing that just to annoy us. When we are in this distortion, we are living in our emotional mind, not our wise mind, and therefore aren't able to see things clearly. This can make us irrational, easily upset, and act in ways that only make us feel worse.

Another distortion is magnification, and this is when we magnify one part of something, ignoring the other equally important components. We could also call this catastrophizing, when we blow things out of proportion.

The next cognitive distortion I want to discuss is labeling, which is when we take one example or experience and judge ourselves or someone else by that, believing that that example is representative of who we are as a person, not just one thing that we did. Let's say we were rude to someone because we hadn't slept well and they were asking a lot of questions; we may tell ourselves we are a rude person, that that's just who we are, instead of thinking that we acted rudely that one time.

One cognitive distortion that I struggle with is "should" statements, where we "should" all over ourselves until we feel terrible about who we are and what we can accomplish. "Should" statements set unattainable high standards and can lead to us feeling that we can't ever measure up.

Finally, there is self-blame. This is when we take responsibility or blame for something we didn't have full control over. I see this frequently in my patients who have been abused or assaulted; they believe that they did something to cause it or that they could have prevented it from happening. Self-blame can erode our sense of self and lead to feelings of shame.

HOW CAN I STOP LIVING IN
THESE COGNITIVE DISTORTIONS?

Once I was able to identify the cognitive distortion that was causing me to constantly apologize, the next step was to restructure it—meaning that I would have to recognize when I was "shoulding" all over myself and force my brain to think about it in a new way. This is, in my experience, the toughest part of CBT work, because we have usually been engaging with this distortion for so long that we don't even notice when we are in it. For me, I always framed my "should" statements as motivational or aspirational, but my therapist helped me to see how often they were sabotaging me. Once I recognized just how hurtful that way of thinking was for me and my life, I was motivated to work to stop it.

One of the ways we can restructure our cognitive distortions is to challenge them with facts or other perspectives. For me, this meant that when I thought something like "I should be doing more with my life," I would force myself to stop and come up with some things that I have already done. For example, I have completed undergrad and graduate school, I have a wonderful and fulfilling job, and I have gotten to travel all over the world. Challenging those false but automatic thoughts helped me see that they weren't true and were only holding me back. If we struggle with a different cognitive distortion, such as all-or-nothing thinking, this would mean that we would have to look for possible middle ground or gray areas. Instead of thinking, "I messed up today, so I might as well just give up completely," we can be softer and look for the things that we did do well, or tell ourselves that tomorrow is a new day and we can start over. The urge to engage with those comfortable false thoughts will still be there, but once we know what our repeat thoughts are, we can recognize and challenge them quickly.

Another way to stop these cognitive distortions from running and ruining our lives is to be curious about them and see how they play out. Now, I don't mean that we should engage with these faulty thoughts and see how much damage they can do, but it can be helpful to see where the thought ends. What I mean by that is, if my thought is "I am going to blow this interview because I should have prepared more," I could let my imagination run through this scenario with the understanding that I won't get the job I am interviewing for, and in the end help me to see that while it's not pleasant or my desired outcome, it's also not life-ending. Letting our brain play out an entire thought or worry can help us to see that it's not worth worrying about and make it easier for us to challenge it or let it go.

While many various CBT techniques are beneficial, the last one that I am going to address is exposure. Once we have recognized our faulty ways of thinking and are fighting to change them, we must practice taking this new action. While it is helpful to role-play in therapy or even visualize ourselves acting in a new, healthier way, we should try it out in our regular life. Continuing to use my example, my exposure had to be completed in busy public places, at work, and home. It started with my not apologizing when someone needed to get past me in a crowded public space, such as the grocery store, yoga studio, or airport. If someone needed to get by, I had to just move (if possible) and say nothing, which sounds simple but was incredibly difficult. Next, if a project took me up until the deadline, I was just supposed to turn it in and not apologize for taking so long. In short, I was supposed to note whether I had done something that made someone else's life more difficult, and if not, I wasn't allowed to apologize. Oh my god, this was so hard.

I also had to try to go for an entire day without apologizing to my husband, Sean (unless I could prove to myself that it was worth apologizing for). This was, by far, the hardest exposure, and I found myself feeling more anxious and unsure than ever before. I would sit in silence trying to consider whether I should apologize for not knowing that the garbage was full and taking it out, or for bumping into him in our very small hallway. I know these thoughts sound crazy, but when you've been saying you're sorry for pretty much everything you have ever done or not done, it can be hard to know what warrants an apology and what doesn't. Over time and with a lot of practice, and checking in with my therapist, I was able to understand that when something I did was upsetting to someone else, it deserved an apology; everything else did not. Sounds simple, but this new way of thinking and behaving took me months to work out, and although I still struggle with this when I am stressed out or upset, it doesn't run my life as it used to.

The interesting thing I learned throughout this process is that I was putting all of this energy into something that did not serve any purpose. My apologizing all the time and feeling that I should have been doing something else didn't help anything, and it didn't improve my life or relationships; it only made me feel bad and less than everyone else. Once I got out of this harmful thought cycle, I was able to see everyday experiences with more clarity, be more thoughtful with my actions, and my life and relationships improved. I realized that a few of my friendships only fed into this unhealthy way of living, and once I wasn't so down on myself or overly apologetic, those relationships didn't work anymore. It was shocking at first, but after deciding to not associate with them anymore, I feel freer and lighter, not to mention it's now easier for me to continue making healthy choices for myself.

WHY IS IT SO HARD TO CHANGE?

While doing some of those CBT techniques can sound pretty simple, in the moment it can be difficult to not engage with the thought, agree with it, and act a certain way as a result. That's why it's important to be kind and compassionate with yourself as you work to make the change. Know that recovery or growth is never a straight line, but more like a winding path with ups and downs along the way. The reason it can be so hard to make these changes is that our brain loves habits, patterns, and consistency, and it will want to go back to what it knows. I have described this in the past as our brain being a balloon filled with sand. Every action we take as a result of how we feel causes a marble to roll across the balloon, creating a small rut to form in the sand, and as we continue to take those actions, that rut will only get deeper. Therefore, when we want to change what has now become our automatic response (the rut we have created), we are going to have to try hard to keep that marble from falling back into that well-worn path.

If we are trying to stop ourselves from getting into yet another abusive relationship, or we want to be out in public without worrying someone is going to hurt us, we are going to have to utilize some of these tools to recognize what cognitive distortions we struggle with most and fight to challenge them. I know it's hard. It's as if we are building a new muscle we never even knew existed, so we can get tired quickly, become frustrated, and want to give up. But stick with it; with each rep, you get stronger and will feel more confident to do it again the next time, and before you know it, a new healthier habit will have formed.

Since we have been talking about learning and how we can change and grow, now is a great time to test your memory. Remember how I told you to spray your favorite scent onto this book and put those three terms into a story so that you can later recall it? What were those three terms? Test your memory, and then take a look back at page 122 to see whether you were right!

HOW DOES THIS RELATE TO TRAUMA?

The reason neuroplasticity and learning are important when it comes to understanding trauma is that they prove we can heal and grow. Too often, when we have been traumatized and are struggling to manage all of the symptoms of PTSD or C-PTSD, we can lose sight of the shore and feel as if we will forever be lost at sea. I hope that this is a reminder of all the research and experience supporting the fact that we can learn new things, and change the way we think, feel, and act. We also have to remember that we cannot change other people or go back in time and prevent the painful experience from occurring; we can only focus on ourselves and the choices we have moving forward. If we don't like how things are going, how we feel, or the relationships we are in, then we have to change something, and it has to start with us.

KEY TAKEAWAYS

- Neuroplasticity is the ability of our brain to adapt and change as we learn things and have new experiences.
- There are three types of behavioral learning: classical conditioning, operant conditioning, and observational learning.
- Classical conditioning is when we pair a neutral stimulus with a naturally occurring response, as Pavlov did with his studies of dogs.
- Operant conditioning is when we use positive or negative reinforcements to increase or decrease a behavior. We can also use punishments as a way of extinguishing a certain behavior, as Skinner did with rats and his "Skinner box."
- Observational learning is when we learn how to do something by watching someone else do it first, as my dogs did when they learned how to let themselves out of their kennel.

- To change our behavior, we have to change our thoughts because they become our feelings, which in turn become our actions. Cognitive behavioral therapy (CBT) works using this principle.

- There are ten cognitive distortions: all-or-nothing thinking, overgeneralizations, discounting positive things that happen, filtering, jumping to conclusions, emotional reasoning, magnification, labeling, "should" statements, and self-blame.

- To change our behavior, we have to track our thoughts, recognize the cognitive distortions that affect us most, and restructure or challenge the distortion. We can also let our imagination play out the thought and expose ourselves to situations that would normally trigger unhealthy behaviors, and try doing the healthier ones.

- By utilizing our ability to learn, change, and grow, we can overcome our past traumas and heal.

CHAPTER 11

THE FOUNDATION OF HEALING

FINDING THE RIGHT TREATMENT

N o matter how hard we try, we cannot forget what happened, and we can't go back in time and make it so that the traumatic situation never occurred. Therefore, the only way to deal with a traumatic experience is to find the right mental health professional and begin working through it. While the style of therapy we enter into is essential, it's more important that we find a therapist we like and have a good rapport with. Doing trauma work can be difficult and triggering, which is why it's necessary that we feel safe with them and in their office. It may take us a few sessions with different therapists before we find a good fit, so don't give up or get discouraged; it's part of the process. Just like dating, on the way to finding someone we enjoy, we usually have to weather a few bad ones first, so stick with it and know that, in time, you will find one that works for you.

One of the ways to know whether you are seeing the right therapist is that you feel they hear you and are on your side. You shouldn't have to keep reminding them of the details about a certain event or the name of an important person in your life; they should take notes and remember. They should also push you to try harder, do a little more than you think you can, and support you along the way. In many ways, a good therapist is like the training wheels on a bike: we may not always need them as we cruise through certain situations, but when things get rough or tricky, they are there to keep us upright and safe. In trauma therapy, faster isn't necessarily better; it can end up causing more pain and upset, and that's why they should challenge us to work through the traumatic events, but not at a pace that's so quick it could be retraumatizing.

Along with finding the right fit in a therapist, we also need to figure out what type of therapy they offer. Not all therapists are trained to do trauma work, and even though their websites may say they do, it's always good to ask them on the phone about it and to specify what types they are trained in. Remember, this is your treatment, time, and money; don't be afraid to make sure they can help you. We wouldn't make an appointment for a heart disorder without first knowing that the doctor is a cardiologist, so why treat our mental health any differently?

WHAT ARE THE TYPES OF TRAUMA THERAPY?

Know that the trauma therapies mentioned are in no way an exhaustive list, nor am I able to include all of the research and data that proves their efficacy. What I hope to illustrate is that there are many options available, and if one isn't working for you, or if you don't have access to some of them, you can still overcome your symptoms of PTSD and heal.

The most common form of trauma therapy is what is known as talk therapy. This means that the therapist will help you put words to what happened, and piece together your experience into a cohesive story. Since most of us have never shared what happened with another person, or even said it out loud before, this process can be daunting and overwhelming at times. However, as we get support and validation for all we have been through, it can also be transformative and healing. It can help us remember what occurred and get us talking about it for possibly the first time, but talk therapy alone isn't always enough. Many of my patients still experience flashbacks or body memories, and feel haunted by what happened. I believe this is because trauma memories are stored differently, and if we can't calm our stress response, we aren't going to be able to piece together what happened any better than we did when it first took place. This is why there are many other forms of trauma therapy out there—if one doesn't work, we can add another or switch over completely.

Another trauma therapy option is eye movement desensitization and reprocessing (EMDR), which was developed by Francine Shapiro in 1988 after she realized that her eyes' tracking people walking past her in the park decreased her response to some upsetting thoughts. She believed that these side-to-side eye movements could potentially help us better manage our negative experiences, or at least lessen the severity of our response to them. Shapiro tried to mimic her eyes' following people walking past by having her patients follow her finger from left to right, and she tested her new treatment and hypothesis on trauma victims. Much to everyone's surprise, she found it to be as effective as exposure therapy and selective serotonin reuptake inhibitors (SSRIs),[1] which was encouraging for many reasons, but especially for people who aren't open to trying medication as part of their treatment.

EMDR is based on the understanding that when something traumatizing happens to us, it overwhelms our system, making it impossible for us to process what took place and neatly file it away into our long-term memory. EMDR gives us another chance to do that at our own pace and allows us to go back to that horrifying experience without being retraumatized by it. When we return to those upsetting images or memories, the EMDR therapist will have you follow their finger with your eyes from side to side, or they may tap you on your left and right shoulders or knees, or even have you hold buzzers that mimic the tapping. I have even been told that some therapists have headphones you can wear that make a beeping noise in your left and right ear separately. All of this tapping and eye movement are used to create bilateral stimulation, which means that we are stimulating both sides of our brain and body and therefore are improving the communication between our brain's hemispheres as well as enhancing our memory.

This style of therapy has been life-changing for many of my patients, some sharing that they didn't even have to talk through all of their trauma memories in EMDR for it to feel less painful. Being able to mentally return to that situation with their new therapeutic resources allowed them to go back to the terrifying experience while still knowing they weren't physically there. They could see what happened from another, more adult perspective, or feel empowered enough to change the way they viewed the outcome. One of my patients told me she could see herself being abused but knew she was an adult now and wasn't going to have to go back there ever again. It allowed her to recognize that the abuse wasn't her fault, and gave her permission to feel angry and sad about what happened. In our previous talk therapy sessions, going back to that time was impossible because she would become so overwhelmed with emotion and feel as if it was happening to her all over again. I referred her to an EMDR therapist and it happened to be just what she needed to finally heal.

In many ways, EMDR sounds like magic, but it's in our ability to return to the memory, feel what happened while knowing we are safe and okay, that it works. Since I can't be inside people's brains while they do it, I can't fully explain why it's effective, but I have seen it transform people, and even though it may sound strange that eye movements could help us heal from trauma, trust me when I tell you it can.

The next style of therapy that can be utilized in trauma work is trauma-focused cognitive behavioral therapy (TF-CBT). This style of therapy was created to specifically help children and adolescents overcome their traumatic experiences, and therefore the parents and caregivers of the child play an active role in the treatment as well. Created by doctors Anthony Mannarino, Judith Cohen, and Esther Deblinger, TF-CBT uses cognitive-behavioral principles and exposure techniques to help alleviate any symptoms of PTSD. The goals with the child or adolescent are to help them understand that how they feel is a normal reaction to trauma, and assist them in building up some ways to self-soothe, relax, and talk themselves down from a trigger or upset. They are also taught to notice when they have fallen into one of the cognitive distortions we discussed in a previous chapter, things like all-or-nothing thinking or catastrophizing. Then, the therapist will slowly expose the child to something triggering and help them to see that that particular object, situation, or smell doesn't have to be scary or traumatizing—they can use their new skills and be okay.[2]

This is where the work with the parents (or caregivers) comes in, as they are supposed to listen to their child as they talk about the trauma and support them so they feel safe and cared for. The adults can only be a part of the therapy if they are not the ones who terrorized their child, and it has been found that having the parents on board for their child's care speeds up their healing process. I would assume this is because the parents can ensure therapy homework is being done, and by their being in session, it can help their child feel more secure to talk about what happened. In some cases, the therapist will even see the parents without the child, to teach them how to model appropriate behavior, when to remind their child to use their relaxation skills, and how to talk about the trauma with their child if they bring it up. I like this style of therapy because it's designed for children and it includes their parents in the process whenever possible. Too often, children don't get the help that they need when they are young and are instead forced to manage their symptoms of PTSD alone, without any skills or understanding of what's going on. Having this type of therapy available gives me hope that more children are being helped and can heal from any trauma they have sustained.

Another type of therapy that can work for anyone who has experienced a trauma in their lives is exposure therapy. This type of therapy is part of cognitive-behavioral therapy (CBT), but I wanted to separate it from CBT to explain why it can be so helpful in healing from trauma. When we are traumatized, we can associate certain smells, sounds, and tastes with that terrifying time, and we work to avoid anything that reminds us of it. This makes sense because if we avoid scary things, then we won't get upset or retraumatized. However, this can make it difficult for us to live our lives and we can feel that we are constantly looking over our shoulder for another person or thing that could hurt us. That's where exposure therapy comes in: It pushes us to encounter these fear-inducing things, work to calm our nervous system down, and prove that it wasn't that scary after all. In a way, we are creating evidence that our amygdala has attached things to our trauma memory that don't belong there, and we are weeding them out one by one.

Just know that exposure therapy doesn't mean you are going to be forced into a scary situation on day one. The first and most important component of exposure therapy is to build up our relaxation skills. We do this first so that when we do expose ourselves to the scary thing, we have some tools to use to help us feel better. Next, we put together a hierarchy of fears, starting with something that is only slightly upsetting, moving up to doing the one thing that is almost too terrifying to consider. When doing the exposures, we will always start at the bottom and work our way up. It's completely fine to skip some of them because they don't seem as scary anymore, or to have to go back and do one over. It's all about going at our own pace and slowly working our way up the list until we get to the top. We can be exposed to these scary things in our imagination, in therapy, or by going to do it ourselves. Whenever I have done this with patients, I usually start by having them imagine they are doing the scary thing, then have them try it in my office (if possible), and finally doing it out in the world by themselves. I find that building up like that lessens the likelihood that they will be retraumatized or get overwhelmed.

The reason I like exposure therapy is that it gives us our life back—the trauma has taken enough already; we don't want it to take away our ability to live our lives and do what we want. It also has an amazing long-term success rate, showing that after four years 90 percent of those treated still had a significant reduction in their fear and impairment.[3]

Another form of therapy that can be beneficial when treating PTSD is somatic experiencing, which was developed by psychologist and trauma specialist Dr. Peter Levine after he noticed that animals in the wild managed the almost daily trauma of their environment by shaking out their body after they had made their way to safety, as a way to regulate their nervous system. This instinctive action expressed all of the energy built up from their fight-or-flight response, and that's why they didn't show any symptoms of PTSD.

This led Dr. Levine to believe that PTSD and its accompanying symptoms are not caused by the trauma itself, but by our nervous system being overloaded by constant perceived life threats. It's because we have all of this energy stuck inside our nervous system that we feel dysregulated, on edge, and exhausted all the time. Therefore, somatic experiencing takes what is called a body first approach: the therapist slowly has you recognize where you feel the trauma in your body and then offers some ways you can move to release it. This style of therapy doesn't focus on recovering memories or putting words to all that's happened; it's more about finding a way to sit with the sensations we have in our body as a result of the trauma, and releasing it. This could be through trembling, doing a full-body shake, or even by taking a trauma-informed yoga class.

I know this sounds a bit odd or silly, but trust me when I tell you I have seen it work. So often, my patients will tell me that they have talked through all of their trauma memories, tried EMDR, and are still having flashbacks or body memories of what happened. Then, they try out a trauma-informed yoga class, and although they are uncomfortable at first, they report feeling less on edge or hypervigilant. I have always believed that if a type of therapy works for one person, then it's worth considering. So before you dismiss this as too new-age for you, consider how you experience your trauma symptoms and whether some therapeutic body movement could be healing.

The final type of therapy I want to address is schema therapy, which was created by Dr. Jeffery Young in the 1980s after he recognized that CBT didn't work as well with his more chronic patients, specifically those who reported unmet emotional needs in childhood. Schema therapy pulls therapeutic techniques from various therapies in hopes of helping people who haven't found much success in therapy thus far. It is based on the belief that when our emotional needs are not met in childhood, we develop these maladaptive schemas to help us survive, but as we get older these schemas get in the way of us using healthy behaviors to get these needs met. These schemas are unhelpful and unhealthy beliefs we have about ourselves and our world, stemming from childhood and continuing into adulthood.

Eighteen different schemas have been identified, but to make it easier to discuss, they have been grouped into five categories. The first category is disconnection and rejection, and this includes such schemas as abandonment and instability, mistrust and abuse, and emotional deprivation. This category of schemas is what can make it difficult for us to develop healthy relationships. If we don't think we can trust anyone, or believe that something is inherently wrong with us so it's best if we are left alone, that doesn't set us up for connection. The next set of schemas are impaired autonomy and performance, which can include feelings of incompetence, enmeshment, fear of harm, and failure. These unhealthy schemas can erode our confidence and make us question our ability to function in the world. The next group is impaired limits, which includes entitlement and superiority as well as lack of self-control or discipline. These schemas can make us competitive, lack empathy for others, and struggle to meet our own goals; even though we can put on a brave face and pretend we are better or more successful than others, we don't honestly believe that to be true. The fourth category is other-directedness, which leads us to put others' needs before ours, ignoring what we think and feel, and doing anything to get the approval of the people around us. This can make it hard to have healthy boundaries, do any form of self-care, or have healthy and balanced relationships. The final group of schemas is known as overvigilance and inhibition, which is when we focus on the negative aspects of life, struggle to express or communicate how we feel, and are hypercritical. This section can make self-reflection or understanding inaccessible, hold us and those around us to impossible standards, and cause us to have grudges for any wrongdoing. These schemas can be incredibly rigid and end up costing us all pleasure or excitement in life.[4]

Identifying the schemas that are alive and well in our life is at the heart of schema therapy. Once we have recognized the ones that affect us the most, we try to see what thoughts and behaviors we have that are reinforcing them. This can be difficult since we have most likely been acting out of these schemas for most of our life, so we need to be patient with ourselves as we force ourselves to think and act differently. Next, we try to figure out where these schemas came from and find other more healthy ways to get our emotional needs met. Throughout this style of therapy, the therapist will try to bring our attention to our schemas as they come up in the therapy session. They will also try to help us see why that way of thinking and acting isn't as helpful as it may feel, and work with us to come up with a new way of interpreting a situation. It may be uncomfortable and slow going at first, but if we can replace these unhealthy beliefs with more balanced thoughts and actions, we will begin to see that the world isn't as scary or hurtful as we once thought. Schema therapy helps us recognize when we are doing something because of what happened to us when we were a child, and challenges us to consider the facts we have now.

I also want to mention group therapy and how beneficial it can be for anyone recovering from a traumatic experience. When we have been hurt by someone, it can be difficult for us to open up to others, and we can even start to believe that what we think and feel is wrong or that we did something to cause the past upset. Hearing from other people who have been through a traumatic situation can help validate our experience, normalize what we have done to try to cope, and get us the social connection we need. Listening to our group member's stories and struggles allows us to offer compassion and understanding, and it can help us see our situation with more clarity and care. There are many benefits to group therapy, but when it comes to trauma work, I cannot recommend it enough, in fact, I believe it should be a required addition to all trauma work.

There are many forms of trauma therapy, and again I just want you to know that if you find one that works for you, stick with it. While therapy itself is never easy, it's always worth it.

WHAT IF THERAPY ISN'T HELPING?

For many people, therapy alone isn't enough. It can feel as though, no matter how many things we try, we can't break free from our symptoms, and that's why there are alternative options. These other treatments do not involve therapy, and although they are completely outside my scope of practice, I felt it necessary to make you aware of them, since it wasn't until this past year that I knew they were an option. The first treatment option is stellate ganglion block (SGB), which is when we get an anesthetic injection to block the growth of the stellate ganglion, a nerve group in our neck that's part of our sympathetic nervous system (responsible for our fight-or-flight response). It is believed that when we are severely traumatized, our sympathetic nervous system is repeatedly activated, causing it to grow extra sprouts of nerves, leading to higher levels of norepinephrine, which in turn activates our amygdala. This is what keeps us held in our PTSD response for long periods, and why no matter what we do, we still feel on edge. By blocking these nerves, we can alleviate the symptoms of PTSD in as little as thirty minutes and the effects can last for years. Researchers believe that this treatment resets our nervous system back to the way it was before we were traumatized. The only thing to consider with SGB is whether we are still involved in a terrorizing situation, and if possible, to wait until we are safe to do the procedure. The SGB procedure has been performed since 1925 and is considered a low-risk pain option with success rates averaging 85 to 90 percent.[5] It began as a treatment to help improve blood flow and manage pain in the neck, head, chest, or arms; however, in 2008, an article was published about its effectiveness in treating PTSD. My only frustration is that this treatment hasn't been more widely tested or known, even though it's been around for almost a hundred years.

Another treatment option for PTSD is vagus nerve stimulation (VNS), whereby a stimulation device is surgically inserted under the skin in our chest that allows an electric impulse to be directed toward our left vagus nerve. Our vagus nerve, also known as the tenth cranial nerve, connects our brain to our peripheral autonomic nervous system (PANS), which is responsible for regulating involuntary bodily functions, such as our heart rate, blood flow, and breathing. During times of trauma or upset, the vagus nerve signals our brain to speed up its storage of memories necessary for survival, and fights against our stress response. In essence, our vagus nerve counteracts our body's fight-or-flight response and helps calm us down so that we can remember key information and survive.[6] Therefore, stimulating our vagus nerve by using VNS can help us calm our system down when we are drowning in our PTSD symptoms.

The final alternative treatment I want to discuss is transcranial magnetic stimulation (TMS), which uses a small electromagnetic coil to stimulate certain areas of the brain, activating the cells in that region and causing them to release neurotransmitters. This small coil does not have to be surgically inserted—it is fixed into a helmet that the patient wears during their treatment—and the magnetic pulses are controlled by a computer program. The patient is awake during the treatment, and although electric pulses are being sent into our brain, it's not painful or felt by most patients. The early TMS studies focused on the prefrontal cortex because of its role in our mood regulation and found that one-hour TMS treatments five days a week for four to six weeks did improve patients' mood.[7] While it is great news that this nonsurgical procedure can help improve our mood and treat such mental illnesses as depression, anxiety, PTSD, and obsessive-compulsive disorder (OCD), it is very time-consuming and therefore not easily accessible. However, it is another potential option for those of us suffering from the symptoms of PTSD.

Another portion of trauma treatment that I want to address is psychotropic medications, such as antidepressants, antipsychotic medications, benzodiazepines, and others. Although the medications themselves do not fully treat PTSD or any mental illness, they do help with some of the symptoms. I am always telling my patients and viewers to think of medication as a life raft: when we are drowning in the symptoms, it can help us get our head above water so that we can take part in therapy. For example, let's say we aren't able to stay present in therapy because we become too overwhelmed and dissociate during each session. Since we know that trauma therapy doesn't work if we are dissociated, medication may help calm our nervous system down so that we can participate and stay grounded in our sessions. I don't believe medication alone can treat PTSD, but it can be part of our overall treatment plan. I am not a doctor; if you are considering medication, you should see a psychiatrist so that you can be assessed and they can decide whether and which medication could work for you. I just think it's important that we know about all possible treatment options so that we can make the decision that's best for us and our healing process.

HOW MUCH TREATMENT DO I NEED?

When it comes to trauma treatment, everyone's needs are going to be different. Some of us will feel good seeing our therapist for one hour a week, whereas others will need to be in an inpatient facility where there is 24-hour support. To help you better gauge whether the level of treatment you're receiving is enough, here is a quick questionnaire:

- Are you able to do all you need to do in your life outside therapy? Able to function at work or at school? In your relationships? Take care of your basic needs?
- When not in session, are you able to manage your PTSD symptoms?
- Do you feel that you can accomplish what you need in your weekly session time?
- Does therapy feel difficult but not impossible?
- Even if it's slow going, do you feel like you are making progress?

If you were able to answer yes to those questions, then the level of treatment you are getting is right for you. Overall, we want to feel challenged in therapy, but not pushed so far that we can't function in our life—meaning we don't want to be so upset by our work in a session that we can't manage the aftermath. Finding that right level of care takes some trial and error, but overall we should feel supported yet pushed along as we heal from all that happened to us.

We all want to get better and overcome our symptoms of PTSD, but unfortunately, trauma treatment is difficult and it takes time. So often, I hear from my viewers how they wish they were moving more quickly through their EMDR sessions or that they just want to get to the point where they feel normal again, and I get it. Having flashbacks, experiencing body memories, and feeling constantly on edge isn't something anyone wants to live with, but healing from trauma is

> Trauma is a fact of life. It does not, however, have to be a life sentence.
> —Peter A. Levine, PhD

one of the times in life when pushing harder and faster won't help us. If we move through it too fast, we can be retraumatized, which can push us deeper into our symptoms of PTSD, and that's why we need moderation and compassion as we slowly make our way. If you are ever feeling lost or like you want to give up, just ask your therapist to run you through some of the progress you have made in your time together; that can help you see how far you have come and all that you have worked through. That's one of the reasons I recommend journaling to most of my patients; having that record of how we were feeling and what we were working on can help us see just how much better things are now, and that can keep us motivated in those dark times when all we want to do is give up. There will be times when we want to give up, or when we don't think it's getting better, but, trust me, every time we fight against the trauma symptoms, we get a little bit stronger and freer.

KEY TAKEAWAYS

- Finding the right therapist is key to doing trauma therapy work. We should feel safe with them, that they listen and are on our side, and that they push us to do more than we think we can.

- There are also many kinds of trauma therapy, and finding the right one for you is important as well. Some popular therapy styles are talk therapy, eye movement desensitization and reprocessing (EMDR), trauma-focused cognitive behavioral therapy (TF-CBT), exposure therapy, somatic experiencing, and schema therapy.

- There are also some alternative treatments if therapy doesn't work for us. These include stellate ganglion block (SGB), vagus nerve stimulation (VNS), and transcranial magnetic stimulation (TMS). Medication can also assist in symptom management.

- Finding the right level of treatment can be tricky, but we should feel challenged yet supported as we work through our trauma experiences.

- Trauma work takes time and effort, so be patient with yourself as you work through it at your own pace. Going too fast can cause us to be retraumatized, which can only worsen our symptoms.

CHAPTER 12

TRIGGERS

HOW TO IDENTIFY
WHAT CAUSES OUR TRAUMA

The word *triggered* has gained more popularity in the past few years, and as with most things, when shared through the telephone game of social media, it loses its real meaning. It has become a joke to many who casually use the term to describe being upset or attacked by something someone said or did. To be triggered isn't a joke or a situation that's merely uncomfortable; it's something in our environment that reminds us of a traumatic event and causes us to have an intense emotional response. This could be a certain smell or sound that we come into contact with and suddenly we are six years old, in that dark room, and being hurt all over again. Many of my patients express how debilitating triggers can be because they can lead to panic attacks, dissociation, or push us into our fight/flight/freeze response. Triggers are things that most people with PTSD avoid at all costs. Although such avoidance can lessen the likelihood of our being retraumatized by our environment, it can also limit what we do in life.

Not knowing what is going to trigger past traumas can make it difficult to decide what to avoid or plan for. This can also make it hard to have relationships, go to work, and live a fulfilling life without feeling constantly on edge. The reason it can be so tough to figure out what's going to upset us is that our nervous system is constantly assessing our environment for any threat, and if we have

> A trigger is something that calls forth a visceral and overwhelming reaction to a stimulus or stimuli that also overwhelms my senses and ability to cope. In other words, I melt.

been traumatized, it is going to connect anything that reminds it of that time to the trauma itself—meaning that even if we were harmed by one man when we were four years old, we can attach everything about that day to the trauma. If we had a snack before the abuse, those food items are now off-limits; or if there was a song playing in the background, we may not be able to listen to anything by that artist without feeling overwhelmed. There is no limit to the number of things that can be triggering to a traumatized person.

These external triggers are often associated with our five senses—what we smelled, touched, saw, heard, or tasted during the terrorizing situation—but they can also be connected to certain dates, times, or places. Some of my patients who had domestic violence in their homes can hear strangers arguing on the street and be thrown into a flashback from their childhood, whereas others struggle around certain trauma anniversaries. Our environment is filled with tons of triggers, which is why PTSD can become so debilitating. If we can't go to our friend's barbecue because they are going to have fireworks and loud noises are triggering, or if we aren't able to go to the mall on the weekends because crowds remind us of our trauma, we can slowly become isolated.

ARE ALL TRIGGERS THINGS IN OUR ENVIRONMENT?

Not all triggers are external or things that we encounter in our environment; for many people, the triggers are internal, such as feeling lonely, out of control, or vulnerable. Just as in the story on the next page, it wasn't the obvious things that triggered her; instead, it was seeing her friend lovingly interact with her children that prompted the upsetting emotional response. We could assume that that was an external trigger because she was watching her friend interact with her children, but I would argue that it's the thoughts and feelings that came up as a result of those interactions that upset her—possibly wishing she had had that type of relationship with her mother or father, or that someone in her life treated her with love and compassion. Whatever it was, it was her thoughts and emotions that ended up triggering her, instead of the overt actions. Internal triggers can be even harder to track down because we don't always know how we feel, especially if we are suffering from PTSD. Being disconnected from how we feel could have been one of the ways we pushed through and survived, because our emotions probably felt overwhelming and not safe to feel for so long.

In my experience, most triggers are both internal and external, but because the external

> Sometimes I will prepare myself for situations and certain triggers, and the things I thought would trigger me were fine, but things I had never even thought about before will trigger me instead. For example, when I am going on a long weekend to visit my friends with small children, I have a plan in place for things that might trigger memories of childhood sexual abuse, like diaper changes, playing dress-up or doctor. But then seeing my friend snuggle her kids, or discipline them with such encouragement and love will trigger me more. Certain very overt things are easier for me to plan for and handle than others. A particular movie was always put in when I was a kid while I waited for my 'turn' for 'special games.' That trigger makes sense to me; it is easy to process and nonconsequential to avoid. Friends being kind to me or their children is harder to understand and much more difficult to not feel ashamed about and I also cannot avoid it if I want friendships.

components are easier to identify and avoid, they are the parts we try to deal with first. It's in the avoidance that these triggers gain more power over us; that's why one of the treatment options I mentioned was exposure therapy. We expose ourselves to something that usually pulls us back into that traumatic memory, but instead of letting it do that, we stay calm and use our therapeutic tools that help prove to our nervous system that that place or thing isn't a threat anymore. It's as though we are giving our brain the chance to double-check whether its belief about that thing is true or false, and by continuing to do this, we build up more evidence that it's not as scary as we thought, which in turn opens us up to more experiences in life without our feeling on edge or disconnected.

Internal triggers, on the other hand, aren't as easy to avoid or expose ourselves to, because we have to figure out what they are first. If we aren't aware of how we are feeling or what it was that upset us about that situation, it can be difficult to deal with or stay away from. Journaling can help, because if we start taking note of the times when we feel overwhelmed or upset, then we can begin to see patterns. Maybe we are always in a situation where someone puts us down, or perhaps being alone for too long causes us to spiral into a dark hole; whatever it is, having it in writing can help us more clearly see the causes. Getting into therapy is the next best step, so that we can talk about these patterns or common situations that elicit our PTSD response. Having a therapist help us tease out what it is about those situations or people that always upset us can help us identify our internal triggers and better manage them.

DO TRIGGERS ALWAYS CAUSE FLASHBACKS?

Triggers are like everything else in psychology: complicated and everyone is going to experience them differently. Not to mention that being triggered isn't always so cut-and-dried: most of us don't only get pulled back into a trauma memory; instead, whatever PTSD symptom we suffer from is followed by the urge to use an unhealthy coping skill, such as under- or overeating, using drugs or alcohol, or engaging in self-injurious behavior. This can make it even more difficult to identify what it was that set us off, especially since a lot of treatment focuses on managing those unhealthy coping skills, not what triggered them. We can spend years trying to get a handle on our drug or alcohol use, but if we aren't able to understand where the urges to use come from, we can be helpless against them.

I had a patient many years ago who, when triggered, would go on shopping sprees, and it took us a while to figure out that it was after she smelled a certain cologne that she started to feel scared and vulnerable. She would feel overwhelmed for a few days and then go on a shopping spree because it seemed to be the only thing that could calm her down. For months, we talked about these shopping sprees, trying to figure out why she engaged in such financially harmful behavior, and it wasn't until a man wearing that cologne got into the elevator with her on her way to my office that we were able to connect the two. Having that understanding allowed us to put together some tools and techniques to help her calm down without spending hundreds or thousands of dollars on things she didn't need.

HOW DO I KNOW WHETHER
I HAVE BEEN TRIGGERED?

We know how easy it is to second-guess ourselves and whether we have been traumatized. From struggling with repressed memories to the feelings of shame that usually accompany any trauma experience, there are so many things working against us. Unfortunately, identifying our triggers can be wrapped up in our ability to recall our past traumas, since they pull from things our brain has connected to the original terrifying experience. However, there are other ways to know whether we have been triggered, and we don't have to fully recall our trauma to be aware of them. First, it's helpful to notice our emotional response to situations in our life and compare our responses to those around us. Let's say we have a terrible boss at work, and she is rude, always publicly calling people out for making mistakes. While everyone in the office hates her and talks badly about her behind her back, they get over it quickly and are only mildly upset. We, on the other hand, may struggle to move past it, feel on edge the rest of the day, and want to file a complaint or quit. If everyone else seems to be only marginally affected by this interaction, there may be more to it for us. It's possible that our boss reminds us of our mother and how she used to yell at us or put us down in front of our friends. Our overreaction is one of the indicators that we may have been triggered.

Another sign is if we have any dissociative symptoms, such as losing track of time or feeling spaced out, unable to snap out of it and pull ourselves back to the present. Although you may think that this is an obvious sign, I find that many of my patients don't even realize they are doing it until I ask them about it. Some of the questions I always ask include: Have you ever driven home and not remembered how you got there? Or felt like you came to while you were doing something? Do you enjoy daydreaming so much you find it difficult to stop when you need to? Often, we don't recognize how checked out we have been unless someone asks us about it, or something else happens while we are dissociated, forcing us back to reality. This urge to check out during our day can be a sign that we have been triggered by something in our environment.

Since avoidance is the easiest way to fend off any possible upsets, noticing whether there are a lot of things we steer clear of is a good indicator of a potential trigger. Especially if other people in our life don't have the same worries or level of discomfort that we do. We all have things we enjoy and don't enjoy doing, and if someone pushed us, we would probably go along with it and be fine, but what I mean are situations that we will not participate in, no matter what. We could even get into arguments with others about it, lying and making up excuses so that we don't have to go. If everyone around us seems to think it's something safe and okay to do, we may be reacting to a trigger from our past.

Since triggers don't only cause us to experience one of the symptoms of PTSD, it's also important to take into consideration the other urges that could coincide with us being triggered. Just like my patient who shopped as a way to cope with smelling cologne, we have to consider other things that we do to manage all we feel. The most common is using drugs or alcohol to numb out from the intense emotional experience, and while it's often socially acceptable to have a drink after work, we may wish we could start drinking earlier or want to drink more than our colleagues. We could also feel this intense urge to exercise or under- or overeat as a response to being triggered. Since our society praises those who exercise regularly, this can go unnoticed for many years until we get injured or we have such a drastic change in our weight that it becomes easily noticeable. I am not saying that having the urge to work out regularly is bad or a sign of being triggered; we just need to distinguish between doing something good for our body versus feeling compelled to do something even if we are sick or injured. My patients who utilize exercise as a way to manage their upsets will go for a run on a sprained ankle or try to work out when they have the flu. These urges are not things we can ignore, and if somehow we are not allowed to do the exercise we need to, we can completely lose our cool. There are many other examples of these types of impulses that can come along with being triggered, such as self-injurious behavior, gambling, porn, or using sex to numb out from the pain or upset. If you find yourself feeling compelled to do something that could later negatively affect you, you may have been triggered.

Finally, along the lines of us having a more intense emotional response than those around us, we could feel overcome with emotion without knowing where it came from. In the first example, I talked about having a mean boss and how that could be triggering because it reminds us of an abusive parent, but sometimes we don't know what initiated the anger or upset we feel. Many of my patients report that their intense emotions seem to come out of nowhere and lead them to act out in ways that are detrimental to their life. We could be going about our day and suddenly feel intensely scared and unable to interact with those around us, or we could be overcome with anger and act aggressively toward others. When we aren't aware of our trauma or haven't had the chance to work through it yet, we can be triggered and have an emotional response to that trigger without being conscious of it. Our inability to track down where these feelings and behaviors came from could be another indicator that we have run into a trigger.

I know it may still be hard to assess whether we have been triggered before, so I have condensed the signs we discussed into this quick questionnaire.

- Do you sometimes have a more intense emotional response than those around you?
- Have you ever lost track of time or have lapses in your memory? Or do you enjoy daydreaming so much it's hard to stop sometimes?
- Do you avoid certain people, places, or things that others don't have issues with?
- Do you suddenly feel the urge to shop, eat, gamble, self-injure, exercise, or use drugs or alcohol? Does that compulsion feel like it comes out of nowhere?
- Do you often feel overcome with emotion and not know why?

If you answered yes to any of those questions, you may have been triggered by something in your environment. Although we may not know much about our trauma or what the trigger was, it is helpful to know whether it's happening to us and to be able to put a name to what we've been feeling. Even though having this information doesn't fully explain what's going on, hopefully it lets us know that how we feel is okay and there is a reason behind it.

IS BEING TRIGGERED BAD?

The reason triggers are something we want to avoid is that it's re-traumatizing to feel thrown back into a terrorizing event. Most of us are not able to distinguish between the actual trauma and a flashback because they can feel the same. This repeated trauma experience can wear away at our self-confidence and our ability to read situations or people. We can start to think that we only cause ourselves more pain because, everywhere we turn, we are hurt again. Since we don't think we can trust ourselves, we can let others make decisions for us, or can be easily pressured into doing something we don't want to do. This can mean we end up engaging in risky behavior that can lead to us being traumatized yet again. In a way, we get caught up in this cycle of traumatized, triggered, traumatized again.

That's why we do all we can to avoid triggers, and if that's not possible, we may use unhealthy coping skills to manage the upset that comes along with it. This has caused many to offer trigger warnings before movies and TV shows, news videos, or posts online, and while I agree that we should warn people before we share something that could be upsetting, I don't think this is always helpful. If these warnings only cause us to remove ourselves from the situation and continue avoiding the thing we fear, we won't get better. The more we avoid these triggering things, the stronger the association will be between these situations and feelings of fear and trauma. It could even cause our brain to connect more things to our trauma, and slowly but surely our world will get very small. That's why I believe trigger warnings only work if we use them to help us gather our tools and therapeutic techniques, and expose ourselves to the situation anyway. I know we won't be able to do that in all circumstances, but we are going to have to challenge ourselves to push against the triggers so that we don't let our past trauma predict our future.

WHY IS IT IMPORTANT TO
KNOW WHAT MY TRIGGERS ARE?

To improve our future, we are going to have to use our triggers to our advantage—meaning that we need to be curious about them, work to identify the things that set us off, and figure out where the fear stems from. They not only tell us what harmed us when we were younger, but also what parts of that we haven't been able to process yet. Triggers bring forth the things we tried to hide away or stuff deep within ourselves, and though they are not comfortable, they are valuable. Since we know they are not rooted in the present, but in the past, our triggers hold the key to our healing. There is this old principle called Chesterton's Fence that comes from G. K. Chesterton's 1929 book *The Thing: Why I Am a Catholic*, in which the author puts forth a pretty simple concept: We should not change something until we first understand what its purpose is. In the book, Chesterton referenced a fence that one man may not see any use for, and therefore he wants to tear it down, but when asked what the purpose of the fence was, he admits that he doesn't know. That man is told to go away and think about why the fence is there, and only once he knows its purpose, can he tear it down.

I believe this principle applies to our triggers and many of our unhealthy coping skills. We can't try to remove them from our life without first understanding what purpose they serve. They exist for a reason, and if we don't acknowledge that reason, these triggers and urges will just keep popping up. I had one patient many years ago who claimed that her eating disorder urges just went away when she moved out of the house and entered college. Sure, most of her stressors came from her having to live with her past abuser, but we had only just begun talking about that, and she was still feeling triggered almost every day. She swore moving out was the answer to her problems, and although I pleaded with her, she stopped seeing me.

About six months later, she called me, very upset, stating that her eating issues had returned and she wasn't sure what she had done wrong. In our sessions together, I learned that she was doing well until she had her first set of finals at college. The stress of having to prepare became too much and she found herself wanting to binge and purge again. I explained that it wasn't anything she had done wrong, but because we hadn't had the time to talk about all her childhood trauma, and better understand what triggered her almost daily, she wasn't prepared for any of life's upsets. In a way, she never understood the purpose behind her eating disorder, and why those urges coincided with times she felt scared and powerless. We hadn't had enough time to get her to see the link between her eating habits and past abuse. Instead, when faced with the stress and pressure of college finals, she used the only coping skill she knew: bingeing and purging.

Know that I wish we could just magically feel better, and moving away from an abusive parent or spouse would just remove any of the scars or triggers from our life, but unfortunately, that's not how our brain works. For us to move past our trauma and heal, we are going to have to work through it, take some time to understand why something is triggering to us, and challenge some of those unhealthy urges. When it comes to trauma work, we can't go over it, we can't go around it, we've gotta go through it.

KEY TAKEAWAYS

- A trigger is something in our environment that reminds us of a traumatic event and causes us to have an intense emotional response.

- There are external and internal triggers. External ones are often associated with our five senses, and the internal ones are connected to our thoughts or feelings about something. Most triggers are both external and internal.

- Ways to know if you have been triggered:

    - Your emotional response is more intense than those around you.
    - You experience dissociative symptoms, such as losing track of time.
    - You find yourself avoiding things other people don't.
    - You have the intense urge to use drugs, alcohol, self-injure, shop, under- or overeat, gamble, or use sex to numb out.
    - You feel emotional and don't know why.

- Being triggered can be retraumatizing, which is why we must learn what causes them, force ourselves to understand where they come from, and get some techniques for better managing them. Avoiding everything that's triggering will only limit what we can do in our life.

- We cannot just ignore or remove our triggers or unhealthy coping skills without first understanding what purpose they serve. They exist for a reason, and until we figure out what that is, they will keep coming back.

CHAPTER 13

BREAKING THE CYCLE

AVOIDING FUTURE TRAUMA & TRIGGERS

I gnoring our triggers doesn't make them go away or help us feel any better; in fact, avoiding them shrinks our world and increases the likelihood of us being traumatized again. That's why we have to find some ways to manage our reaction until we can get them to go away for good. The tools and techniques that help get us through any upset are called coping skills. Coping skills, by definition, enhance our ability to adapt to our environment—meaning that they ready us for anything life can toss our way. Building these skills will be vital, as they allow us to expose ourselves to some triggering things and not be overcome with PTSD symptoms. In short, our coping skills will help us get our life back to what it was before we were traumatized.

As we discussed, exposure therapy is best for dealing with triggers, though it's uncomfortable and probably the last thing any of us want to do. This style of therapy involves building up coping skills to deal with the anxiety and upset that triggers bring, and then slowly exposing ourselves to the triggering thing. It can be difficult, and we can still get upset or feel anxious, but for us to move on, heal, and live a full life, we have to challenge our trauma beliefs. Our brain has connected all of these things to our trauma, and it will continue to add more if we don't challenge it. That's why building up these skills, and walking toward our triggers, is key to healing and moving on, not to mention that exposure therapy is highly successful and rarely has to be repeated.[1]

WHAT IF I DON'T KNOW
WHEN I AM BEING TRIGGERED?

The first step is to learn some mindfulness skills so that we can tell when we are upset versus calm. I know that can sound silly, and you may think it's easy to tell, and if so, you can skip on to the next section. However, many of us struggle to recognize when we are triggered or upset, and therefore it can be hard to know when we need to use these coping skills and for how long. My favorite mindfulness technique is what I call 4x4 breathing, when we breathe in for four seconds, hold it in for four seconds, and breathe out for four seconds, and we do this four times. It's pretty simple, we can do it anywhere, and it can help calm our nervous system down. For this breathing technique to be a mindfulness skill, we have to focus on where we feel the breath: think about how it feels on the edge of your nose, how it fills up your belly, chest, or shoulders, and the release you get from breathing out. Pulling our attention to what's happening inside our body can help us better recognize when we feel tense, or are not breathing deeply, and do something to cope with it quickly.

The next mindfulness technique I frequently use is to start identifying our emotions. Too often, we don't even recognize what it is we are thinking or feeling, which can cause us to be in pain for longer than we have to. I love feeling charts for this, and you can easily search for them online; they are just lists of emotion words, and you can print them out and start circling two or three each day. Some of my patients can easily recognize what emotions they are experiencing without the charts, but I find that seeing the feeling words written out already can help us decide what it is we feel and possibly even unearth an emotion we were trying to stuff down. I have my patients try to do this every day, working up to identifying five every time they do it. It may sound difficult at first, but with time and practice, it does get easier.

While there are many other mindfulness techniques out there, those are the ones I work on first before moving on to coping skills. Having the ability to tap into how we feel and recognize when our body is tense and dysregulated will help us know when to use our coping skills and even help us pick out which one we should use in the moment.

Next, we need to come up with some coping skills that help us feel soothed and okay. Everyone's are going to be different, so don't think that just because someone said they love breathing exercises that you have to agree; pick some tools that help calm you when you are feeling overwhelmed. I like to break these coping skills into two buckets: those that help us process what we are feeling, and ones that help distract us from the painful thoughts or experiences. The reason I do this is that there are going to be times when we can't focus enough to process all we are feeling, but we still need to deal with the flashbacks or other PTSD symptoms. There will also be times when we need to pinpoint what it is we are feeling and consider why that's so triggering. Each of these instances will call for specific types of coping skills; therefore, to handle anything life throws at us, we need to have tools for both instances.

WHAT IF I CAN'T PROCESS ALL I AM FEELING?

Let's start with the distraction-based coping skills, since these are the ones we can most easily engage in when we first start to deal with our past trauma. When we are triggered, we may not have the ability to process anything in the moment; we just need a break from the terrible

I try to limit the amount of time I think about it outside of my therapy sessions with distractions. I use music, reading, movies, pretty much anything but silence to keep my mind from thinking about it. Time also helps.

feeling, and that's where these coping skills come in. One of the easiest ways to distract our mind is to move our body; we can do this by stretching, going for a walk, or even joining a workout class. Exercise releases endorphins, chemicals that lessen our ability to feel pain and make us feel good, which is just an added benefit while getting our mind off what's upsetting us.[2] Also, remember that movement is a cornerstone of somatic experiencing therapy and what Dr. Levine has based his life's work on, so getting out and exercising has many benefits when it comes to our trauma treatment.

I regularly recommend going for a walk to my patients and viewers, not only because of the benefits we just discussed, but it also gets us away from any trigger or unhealthy coping skill. If we tend to abuse alcohol or drugs, engage in self-injurious behavior, or over-shop online, getting out of the house limits our access to the items we use in our harmful behavior. This can allow us to breathe, consider our options, and make a better decision.

Another helpful distraction technique is doing a craft, such as coloring, painting, or doodling. As we get older, we tend to stop doing crafts, but it can help to have some on hand for when we are triggered or have a bad day. Pulling our focus off of the upsetting event and onto staying in the lines or drawing mountains with snowy peaks can help us ride the wave of emotion without getting pulled under.

One of the coping skills we saw in full effect when COVID-19 first hit was cleaning or organizing our house. This is not only a great way to keep our hands and mind busy, but it can also give us a sense of accomplishment and make us feel more comfortable in our space. As I said at the beginning, not every skill is going to work for you, so pick and choose whatever you like, kind of like a coping skill buffet.

Now I could go on and on with ideas for distractions, such as bowling bubbles and imagining our issues are the bubbles and we watch them burst and disappear, but you get the idea. A distraction coping skill helps us focus on something else for the time being until we feel calm enough to process why we felt that way or expose ourselves to the scary thing once again.

Before we move into the process type of coping skills, I want to add one thing that I believe belongs on both the distraction and process lists, and that is supportive people. The reason I think they straddle both styles is because we can choose to share what we are going through or not, but either way, they are helpful and soothing to our system. We can even have people we only reach out to because they love to talk about themselves, and that can be a nice and much-needed distraction. We can also have people we are close to who will know we are upset from the moment they hear our voice and want to know what's going on and how to help. Both types of people are helpful and should be on our list of possible ways to cope. We know how important connection is to our nervous system and that it's the true antidote to our stress response, so working on this list will be a vital part of our trauma recovery. We can also benefit from being around animals, whether we foster, adopt, or even volunteer at a local shelter. They can give us a reason to get up and out each day, and remind us that we are not alone. It can also help to know that someone is depending on us for their survival, and that can give us purpose and motivation when it may otherwise be hard to come by.

HOW TO TURN A TRIGGER
INTO A THERAPEUTIC RESOURCE

Distracting ourselves from how we feel will only get us so far because it doesn't help us understand or process what we are going through; it just gives us something else to focus on for a while until the intense feelings or flashbacks pass. Once those emotions have passed and we are feeling calmer, we are going to have to utilize some process-based coping skills. These are the tools we will use to make sense of what has happened to us, help us better understand why we are feeling this way, and gain a new perspective and insight on the issue. They are a bit more intensive and will require us to slow our thinking down so that we can consider a different emotional response.

My most utilized process-based coping skill is impulse logs. These are things we fill out whenever we feel the urge to abuse alcohol or drugs, engage in self-injurious behavior, or really do anything that could harm us and those around us. They help us recognize how we are feeling, what we can do instead, and increase our tolerance for intense emotion. The reason I use impulse logs so often is that they help create time and space for us to make positive decisions, rather than be driven by our emotional impulses. These logs are lifesaving and could be the difference between our staying sober and falling off the wagon or even the reason we don't self-injure when upset. I could attempt to explain what an impulse log is, but it's easier to share one with you so that you can create your own and use them as needed. The one that I use most was created by S.A.F.E. ALTER-NATIVES, which is an organization that offers treatment for those

Impulsive/ self-destructive thoughts	Day and time	Where are you?	What's the situation?	What feelings are you having?
Ex. I am broken and cannot be fixed. I should just drink until I can't think about it.	Tuesday at 10pm	At home	My friend asked me why I am not better yet, and why I still go to therapy twice a week	Judged, sad, mad, shameful, disgusted, and anxious

suffering from self-injurious behaviors, as well as training for clinicians.[3] While its focus is on treating self-injury, I believe this impulse log can be used to manage any unhealthy impulse we may have. I have added an example to help you better understand the nine different columns.

I know doing these logs can seem tedious and frustrating at times, but stick with it. As we do more and more of these, we can start to see patterns in our thoughts and behaviors. Maybe we tend to be triggered when we are around certain people, or are more vulnerable to things during a specific time of year. As I mentioned previously, all of that information is helpful when we are trying to manage our triggers, because the more we know about what triggers us the better we can prepare for it.

Another less structured way to begin processing is to journal, and no, journaling doesn't have to be like keeping a diary, and we don't have to write about everything that happened each day. Journaling is just a way to keep track of how we feel, to note what's going on that could be upsetting us, and to push us to think of some things we are looking forward to. The goal of journaling is to get some of what we are worrying about out of our head and onto paper, so that

Result of doing the impulsive thing?	What are you trying to communicate with this behavior?	What action did you take?	What was the outcome?
Breaking my sobriety, I would have to tell my sponsor, I'd feel embarrassed, and like I threw away my progress.	That I am doing the best I can and I need more understanding and support.	I called my sponsor and texted with my therapist.	The feelings passed and I am glad I didn't drink. I am even kind of proud of myself.

we can put words to what's going on and gain a new perspective on it. This can also help when we are feeling stuck in therapy or that we aren't making enough progress; by journaling regularly, we can look back a few months and see how much we have changed and grown.

If even the idea of journaling is overwhelming and makes you want to give up, just try writing out your answers to these three questions every day for one week and see whether it helps: What's one thing you are grateful for? One thing you are working on? And finally, what is one thing you are looking forward to? We can also write letters to those who hurt us and then rip them up or safely burn them, without sending them. This can be another way to express what we are going through without feeling that we are writing in a diary or have to document everything that happens each day. One thing I will recommend you do if you choose to write letters to those who harmed you is to also write a letter to someone you love and care for. Taking the time to shift our mind away from the pain and onto how much someone means to us helps prevent us from thinking all people are terrible and out to get us. It can be a much-needed reminder that people do care, we are loved, and there is support available to us.

The final process-focused coping skill I want to talk about is creating a feeling word collage. I know crafting seems like something only children do, but trust me when I tell you that this can help people of all ages recognize the emotions they are having when all they want to do is shut down completely. The way feeling word collages work is you start with one emotion you want to work on: write it out in big letters in the middle of a piece of paper. Feel free to use block letters or even color in the word with a shade that you feel fits that emotion. Next, begin to add other words that connect with that feeling until you have filled up the rest of the paper. In case that wasn't very clear, let's say we are working on the feeling of anger; I would write ANGER in big letters in the middle of my sheet of paper and then add other words around it, such as *mad, tense, impulsive,* or *scared.* Doing this for emotions that are difficult to understand or process can help us see how we experience the feeling and possibly what caused it. It can help us untangle all the swirling thoughts and emotions so we can more clearly see our process. Also know that it is very common to struggle with emotions that are seen as positive, just as much as with the more negative ones; what's important is that we select the feeling words that are uncomfortable to us.

WHAT IF COPING SKILLS DON'T HELP ME?

Too often, distraction- and processing-based coping skills don't help my patients when they are struggling with trauma triggers, and that's why we also utilize grounding techniques and safe spaces. We discussed grounding techniques a few chapters back when we were learning about dissociation, but they can also assist us when we are trying to stave off a flashback or other PTSD response. These can include counting the number of things in the room that are blue or green, as well as eating "hot" candy or smelling something with a strong scent. Using our five senses to bring us back into our body, instead of letting the trigger take us back to the trauma, can save us from being upset all over again.

Consider how you can use your five senses to keep you present and make sure you always have some tools on hand so you are prepared for any potential trigger. For example, if smells can be triggering, maybe we keep a bottle of peppermint essential oil with us to sniff quickly before the other scent pulls us into a flashback. Or perhaps we keep cinnamon candies in our backpack or purse, so that we can pop one in if we start to feel overwhelmed or spaced out. Try out a few different tools and techniques, and when one works, make sure you have access to it at all times.

If we aren't able to use our senses to keep us present and calm us down, we can also use our imagination and go to a safe space.

Safe spaces are places we can go in our imagination that help us feel protected and okay. This could be the home of someone who always defended us, the apartment we lived in before the trauma, or a space we have created in our mind that helps us feel peaceful. Whenever I feel overwhelmed or stressed out, I imagine myself floating in the ocean off the coast of Costa Rica, my ears below the surface of the water, quieting any outside noise, and the sun hot on the bits of my skin exposed to the sun as I feel the waves rock me from side to side. That was one of the most relaxing and peaceful times of my life, and taking myself there in my mind stops any thoughts, feelings, or impulses from ruining my day. Take some time to remember or create some of your own; just make sure these places feel safe and secure so that when you go there, you know you are okay.

HOW DO I TALK TO PEOPLE ABOUT MY TRIGGERS?

Whenever we are struggling, we must share what's going on with those in our lives. We don't have to tell everyone we know about our trauma and what we are doing to manage it; however, we do need to find a way to communicate with those closest to us. They need to know what we are working on, how it can affect them, and what they can do to help. That way, if we are having a bad day, they don't jump to conclusions and assume it's something they did or didn't do; instead they can check in or realize it's because of what we are personally working on.

Before we share anything about our trauma experience and treatment with those around us, consider what it is we are comfortable with their knowing and try to break it down into a maximum of three to five points. This can help us stay on track, not dump everything at once, and ensure that we share what we need them to know. For example, one bullet point could be:

- *I have some stuff that happened to me in my past and I am working through it, but it's causing me to be on edge and more easily upset. I wanted to tell you so you know that it has nothing to do with you.*

We will also want to let them know of any indicators that we are being triggered or having a flashback, and whether there is something they can do to help. This can give us another layer of support so that if we aren't able to help ourselves, someone else can be there to comfort us and get us through. Additionally, it's helpful to figure out what we need from them, and add that after the three to five bullet points. We could ask for support and check-ins, see whether they can help us pay for therapy or other appointments, or maybe give us a ride to and from our consultations. It is going to differ depending on how and where we engage with them. If we work together, we may want them to sit next to us in meetings, or bring us a hot drink before we have a presentation; and if we live together, we may need them to give us space or help us get to our appointments. Consider how they could assist you best, and make sure you ask for the help. I know it's difficult to ask others to do things for us, but if the roles were reversed, I know that we would want to know how to help them. Allow them to support you when you need it most.

Finally, we need to make time for this conversation, and do it when we aren't already maxed out or in a rush. We want everyone involved in the conversation to be present and able to hear what we have to say. Don't try to talk about sensitive issues during a holiday meal or an argument. Wait until things are less intense to let them know what's going on, and also remember that we don't have to say everything about the issue in one conversation. This is the first of many discussions, so if you don't get it all out, don't feel pressure to fit it in; you can always bring this topic up at another time. We have to give our loved ones time to digest what we are telling them, and hopefully, they will come back to us with questions as well as the type of support we asked for.

As we work to better manage our triggers, and expose ourselves to things we thought were scary only to realize they aren't that bad, we will slowly learn to trust ourselves again. We can start to feel more confident in our decision-making skills, and in our ability to ride out the ups and downs of life. This newfound trust in ourselves can make us less likely to be traumatized again, whether it's from triggers in our environment or new experiences. As we feel stronger, we will be able to more quickly recognize detrimental behavior, develop healthy relationships, and finally feel in control of our life and future. Doing this work is difficult and exhausting at times, but our trauma has already taken so much from us, I think it's time we took back what is ours.

KEY TAKEAWAYS

- Ignoring our triggers will only make them stronger. Using exposure therapy to help us realize that what we thought was scary wasn't that bad is how we heal and move past our trauma.

- To engage in exposure therapy, we have to have coping skills to help us calm our nervous system down while we are exposed to the trigger.

- For us to know whether we have been triggered, we have to be able to tap into our body and how it feels. Using 4x4 breathing can help us calm down, and allows us to identify some of the emotions we feel each day.

- One style of coping skill is distraction, such as going for a walk or exercising, coloring or other arts and crafts, as well as cleaning and organizing.

- Once our nervous system is calmer, we can engage in the process-based coping skills, such as journaling and using our impulse logs. This can help us acknowledge and gain perspective on all we are feeling.

- If distracting and processing coping skills don't work, we can always use grounding techniques, such as smelling a strong scent or going to a safe space in our imagination. We can also revisit a pleasant memory.

- We have to talk to our loved ones about our trauma, triggers, and what we are working on. This allows them to support us and can help them understand why we may be having a tough time or are acting out.

CHAPTER 14

RESILIENCE

BUILDING IT & KEEPING IT

*R*esilience is defined as our ability to cope with emotional distress and know that we will be okay. Another way to describe it would be our capacity to bounce back after something bad happens to us, and when healing from a traumatic experience, resilience is what keeps us going. Resilient people can reach out for support when they need it, meet the demands of work or school, and know when they need to take a break. Resilience isn't something you can achieve once and use for a lifetime; it is something we constantly have to work on, and depending on our current state we may have more or less of it.

Many years ago, I took a continuing education course focused on working with teens in a school setting. I had hoped to learn how to help them regulate their emotions and communicate with them in the best ways, in order to ensure that if I decided to work in the school system, I could be effective at my job. Although I did learn a lot during that session, what I walked away with was what the course instructor called the poker chip analogy: that when we wake up in the morning, we all have a certain number of poker chips in our bag. We could have ten, or maybe five depending on how well we slept and whether we are sick or we are dealing with some emotional pain. When we are getting ready for our day, let's say we receive a text from a colleague telling us they won't be there for our presentation together; well, that stress is going to cost us two poker chips. We go to make our coffee and realize we are out of beans—toss one more poker chip in the pile. Then, we get on the freeway to head to work and there's a traffic jam—that's going to cost us yet another poker chip. For many of us, by the time we get anywhere, we could be out of poker chips, which means that when we encounter another stressful or upsetting situation, we can't just toss out another chip and move on; instead we can lash out, lose our cool, and feel completely out of control. The poker chips that we had are our built-up resilience, and the more of it we have, the better we will be able to get through life without acting in ways that only leave us feeling worse. We want to build up extra so that on those particularly difficult days, we can dig deep into our bag and pull out the chips we need.

ARE SOME PEOPLE BORN WITH MORE POKER CHIPS THAN OTHERS?

On the one hand, I believe we are all born with a certain amount of resilience; for example, some of us are more resourceful, outgoing, or intuitive, any of which can give us more ways to cope with something terrible instead of being wiped out by it. On the other hand, many people are shy, struggle to make new friends, and prefer to numb out from all they feel. This discrepancy would explain why one sibling can come out of an abusive home struggling with addiction and self-hatred, while another can focus on school, build a support system, and move on successfully. It's also important to mention that our parents are often the first examples of resilience, and if they modeled the use of positive coping skills and resources, then we will have a leg up on those whose parents didn't. Also, some of us may have better access to resources like group activities or supportive family or friends, which will make building up our resilience easier as well. Now, that doesn't mean that only some of us will be able to recover, it just means that we may have to work a bit harder to build up our resilience, which is why it's important to show yourself a little compassion as you get started.

HOW DO I BUILD MY RESILIENCE?

Building resilience starts with our ability to take care of ourselves; we can't deal with something hurtful or stressful if we didn't get enough sleep the night before. Not to mention, the word *hangry* exists in our vernacular for a reason: when we haven't eaten in a while, we can be more irritable and impatient as opposed to how we act when we have a full stomach. That's why one of my favorite dialectical behavior therapy (DBT) tools is HALT. It stands for "hungry, angry, lonely, tired." We are supposed to "halt" and check in on those things before making a decision or engaging with someone.[1] This can tell us whether we are in a position to think things through with a clear mind or if we are filled with impulsive and emotional thoughts.

By ensuring we eat regularly, process our anger, connect with loved ones, and get enough sleep, we are lowering our vulnerability to our environment and emotions. This also increases our ability to cope with all we feel and still make positive, helpful decisions, which is, you guessed it, what resilience looks like. This simple acronym HALT can help us slow down our reactions and ensure that when we engage with others we are doing so thoughtfully and with care, instead of acting impetuously.

It's also important that we recognize when we need to take a break from something. This could be a difficult project at work, a relationship we are in, or even when we need to rest and do nothing. Although this seems like something we should all realize, it can be hard to know when we have had enough, and if I'm being honest, I struggle with this one the most. It's hard for me to notice when I am overworking myself, feeling burned out, or putting too much energy into something and need to stop. Therefore, I often find myself feeling completely drained. I think we struggle to recognize when enough is enough because we don't check in on ourselves regularly. Instead, we compare ourselves to other people who are doing better than us and ignore the signs that we may be physically or emotionally worn out. Being mindful of how we feel, and noting the evidence that we are tired or overworked, is important and a huge component in building up our resilience.

Going back to something we discussed in previous chapters, connection helps calm our stress response and therefore is vital to our resilience as well. Although casual relationships have their benefits, deeper understanding offers more support and the necessary reminder that we are not alone in our struggles. Feeling that other people care about us is life-affirming and gives us someone to reach out to when we need help. Recovery from our past trauma is hard and we are going to need other people outside of ourselves to lean on when we can't stand on our own. Having this true connection also allows us to offer support when someone needs it, which can give us a sense of purpose and meaning. Which, you guessed it, helps us build even more resilience.

Finding social support is often the most difficult task for my patients because if we have suffered from PTSD symptoms for a long time, we could have isolated ourselves so that we don't get triggered or retraumatized. Many have told me how they stopped replying to texts, not calling people back or going to parties, and now don't feel that they have anyone they can count on. If you find yourself in a

> **"** When I was traumatized, my relationships were my stability. Trauma can steal away many facets of your sense of self and I found myself terrified I wasn't going to be me ever again. It's like you're swimming in the depths of the pool and someone guides you to the top and reminds you to breathe some fresh air. That fresh air is what keeps you going.

similar situation, don't fret; there are some simple ways to get you reconnected and feeling better. First, if you had a healthy relationship with someone before, it's okay to reach back out. Sure, it's been a while, but all you have to do is acknowledge that you stopped responding and hanging out, and let them know why. Then, check in: Ask how they are and whether you can get together in the next couple of weeks. I know the thought of reaching out can be hard, but what have you got to lose? If they don't reply or aren't interested in getting reconnected, you are right back where you are now, so send that text! Do it now! Start building up that social support one message at a time.

If you didn't have any healthy past relationships, it may take more effort, but asking your therapist whether they know about or offer group therapy sessions is a great place to start. Also, finding groups online can give us some extra support, as well as many of the peer support sites, such as TalkLife, 7 Cups, and Crisis Text Line. If those options don't render any results, you can join a gym or workout studio, a church, or even take group music lessons. Finding an activity we enjoy and doing it with other people makes it easy to strike up a conversation, get to know people slowly, and decide whether we want to pursue that relationship. To meet new people and build up our support system, we are going to have to say yes to some new social activities. I know it can be uncomfortable, but through discomfort comes growth and resilience.

One of the traits that all resilient people have is a belief in their ability to change and grow. We just have to know that we can change and grow, and believe in that. The shift in our thinking is subtle but important because when grappling with PTSD, we can struggle with shame, guilt, and embarrassment, making confidence hard to come by. Therefore, it can be easier to agree that we do have choices and that there are things we can do to help us adjust and manage our life. Making that shift can cause us to feel more empowered and motivated, which—you guessed it—builds more resilience.

Although making that small shift in our thinking can sound easy, it's often difficult and can require us to pay attention to the thoughts and beliefs that consistently run in our mind, and work to make them more positive. This doesn't mean we have to only think positive things, but instead of allowing our brain to get caught in a shame spiral, we can reframe the thoughts. Reframing is when we consider and then create a new way of looking at something. We can do this with our thoughts and beliefs, and an easy way to find out whether we need to reframe them is to answer these four questions:

- Did we use absolutes, such as *always, never, nobody,* or *everybody*?
- Are we engaging in blaming language?
- Are we shouldering all responsibility for a situation that involved multiple people?
- Do we think we can read people's mind or see the future?

If we said yes to any of those questions, we are going to want to reframe our thoughts—meaning that we will need to consider an alternate perspective. For example, is it possible that we don't always upset people? Or maybe we aren't the only ones to blame for a bad experience? Are we open to the idea that we don't know all the facts, and therefore cannot be sure something is going to turn out badly? When we are using absolutes and other unhelpful thought traps, they don't leave us open to the belief that we can make better choices and that things could turn out okay. If we find it difficult to consider the possibility of a better future, notice whether we are falling into one of those traps, and fight back by reframing the thought. This can help us see opportunities for growth and have a more balanced outlook on our life.

Another way I help my patients reframe their struggles or automatic thoughts is through natural curiosity. Before we jump to judge ourselves for a decision we made or an issue we are having, could we be curious about it? Maybe we could try to learn more about the situation or strive to understand our response. Wanting to know more about ourselves and the reasons behind our actions can keep judgment at bay and give us helpful information about ourselves and our past. If we feel uncomfortable when our friend tells us how grateful they are for us, can we attach that reaction to something from our past? Maybe we can try to search our memory for a time when someone complimented us, only to harm us afterward? Or perhaps whenever we are told we are helpful and kind, we worry that we can't live up to it and our self-doubt and shame get in the way. Being curious about the reasons we think and act as we do allows us to learn about our experience without punishment or penalty, and the more we know, the better able we will be to change and grow.

If we are still finding it difficult to believe that we can adapt and develop, journaling can be another helpful tool. Keeping track of what we are struggling with, working on, and looking forward to can help us get everything out of our head and onto paper (or our computer). This prevents us from ruminating on past events or focusing only on the negative things, but it's also helpful when building up our resilience. After we have been journaling for a bit, we can look back on our frame of mind from a week or even a year ago and see how much we have changed. It can prove to us that emotions and upsets pass, as well as show us just how far we have come on our path to recovery. When we are having a bad day or struggling with the symptoms of PTSD, it can feel as though it will never get better, but having proof that it already has can keep us motivated and believing in our abilities.

WHAT IF I AM TOO DAMAGED?

Too often, I hear from my patients and viewers that they don't believe they can get better, that they are broken, or too far gone. While this experience can feel incredibly real at the moment, know that it's not true; it's just shame lying to us and stealing our belief in our ability to change. Shame likes to hold us captive, push us down, and make us think something is innately wrong with us. This is why we have to fight back, push against the shame, and overcome the fear it feeds on, and the first step in doing that is using bridge statements.

Bridge statements are phrases we use to move our negative thoughts into a more positive place. These aren't outright positive statements, but they do help build a bridge toward a more positive place, and they apply here as well because shame isn't something we can just ignore or push past easily. We are going to have to slowly shift our beliefs about ourselves one thought at a time—meaning that we will need to start tracking those automatic thoughts and actions. Before you jump to conclusions, know that you don't have to keep track of every thought you have each day. Just start paying attention to what you say to yourself about how you relate to others, how well you can do things in life, and how you feel about yourself and your abilities. Keep track of these because it's likely that you are having the same five to ten thoughts relating to you and your worth over and over again. These repetitive thoughts are holding you in your shame and trauma experience, and recognizing them is the first step in getting them to go away.

Once we have narrowed it down to these repeat offenders, let's try to make them less shame filled. For example, instead of thinking that we are too broken to get help, could we think that while we are broken, someone may be able to assist us? It may not work, but we could feel a bit better or at least have someone who will listen to us. I know that doesn't seem like a big shift, but that's okay; that's the point of bridge statements, to help us move slightly closer to a more positive outlook. Each time we have those automatic and shame-filled thoughts, let's try to shift them into the "maybe," "possibly," or "I am open to" type of thoughts. Not taking our shame thoughts at face value allows us to show ourselves some compassion and consider another perspective.

This type of work is hard, and it can be exhausting at times, but just being more aware is a huge step in the right direction. Too often, we are asleep at the wheel, letting our thoughts flutter in, accepting them as facts, and acting in harmful ways as a result. Being more conscious of what we allow ourselves to think and believe helps us weed out any false facts and unhealthy thought traps, leaving space for logical thoughts and choices. It can also prevent us from quickly jumping into a shame spiral or numbing out completely, such as when someone offers some constructive criticism about something we did and we immediately feel a pit in our stomach and consider all the ways we messed up in our life, or when we lash out in a rage when someone offers us another perspective. These are all signs that we are not acknowledging our feelings of shame and challenging them, and the more aware we become, the less power it will have over us.

It can also help to separate who we are from what we do. Just because I am a therapist doesn't mean that that's all there is to know about me; I am a complex person with many hobbies, beliefs, and ideas, and you are too. Taking a handful of experiences and choices we have made and believing that that is representative of all we can be isn't right. We go through phases in life, we grow and change, and the choices I made when I was younger are not the same ones I would make today, and that's okay. Notice when shame tries to focus on only a few of those past choices and push you to believe that they are indicative of who you are as a whole. When we feel that urge, recognize it for what it is, a lie, and choose to focus on some of the good things we have done. If we aren't able to come up with any good things, it can also help to focus on the things we did that weren't good or bad, but just okay. At the very least this can help us have a more balanced outlook on our lives and our decision-making skills instead of being pulled into an all-or-nothing, shame-filled thought process.

As we work through this, just remember that we are all allowed to be less than perfect. We don't always act appropriately or make the best decisions, but that doesn't make us bad people; that makes us human. It can even help to write this reminder on sticky notes and put them all over your house so that you don't forget, because if we let that message allude us, shame will jump right back in and get cozy, and that's not what we want. We want to accept that mistakes happen, and we aren't perfect, but we can learn and grow for a better tomorrow.

WHY DO I NEED RESILIENCE?

When we start trying to build our resilience, it can feel like an insurmountable task, and we can try to find shortcuts or easier ways to cope, but we need to stay the course. Resilience is vital to our growth and healing because it prevents us from being traumatized again by minimizing the potential for us to be pushed into our stress response. As our resilient zone gets larger, it moves in on the areas that used to be utilized for our fight/flight/freeze response, which gives us more opportunities to ride out the waves of life without being overwhelmed by them. Think of life as a wavy line running along a sheet of paper, and as stressful things occur, it moves closer to the top or bottom of the sheet. The middle section of this piece of paper is our resilient zone, and the top is fight and flight, while the bottom is our freeze state. Doing this work slowly grows that middle section—meaning that we can ride out more intense ups and downs more easily, use our skills, and stay present. This will help us be less vulnerable to triggers, and even allow us to do more trauma work in therapy.

Think of this resilient zone as our poker chip bag, and as we build it up, that bag expands to house all of the skills and techniques needed to weather the storm. We want to take any opportunity to add to that bag, which means that even if we are only able to add one more poker chip to our bag this week, that's amazing progress and gives us the ability to manage one more upset than we could before. Paying attention to these incremental gains will help keep us motivated, more positive, and end up adding more poker chips to our bag than we originally thought possible. Before we know it, we will be able to handle any trigger or difficulty while remaining calm and clearheaded.

KEY TAKEAWAYS

- Resilience—our ability to cope with emotional distress and know that we will be okay—is important in trauma recovery.
- Some people have more resilience than others because of their personality, ability to reach out for support, or their parents' modeling resilient behavior.
- We can build resilience in the following ways:

  - Taking care of our basic needs and checking in to make sure we aren't hungry, angry, lonely, or tired (HALT).
  - Knowing when we need to take a break.
  - Growing our social support system.
  - Focusing on our ability to change and grow.
  - Reframing any negative or unhelpful thoughts.
  - By being curious about our progress and decisions instead of judging them.
  - Journaling can also help us keep track of our progress.

- Shame is the belief that something is innately wrong with us, and it can try to impede our recovery.
- We can fight back against shame by doing these few things:

  - Use bridge statements to argue against the shame thoughts.
  - Separate who we are from what we do.
  - Remember that no one is perfect and making mistakes is part of being human.

- We need to build up our resilience so that we are less and less likely to be pushed into our fight/flight/freeze response while working to process our past traumatic experiences.

CHAPTER 15

BUILDING SUPPORT

HOW TO HAVE HEALTHY RELATIONSHIPS

S upport is necessary when working to overcome any traumatic experience. Unfortunately, trauma doesn't only affect those who are personally harmed by it; the ripple effect of trauma can be felt by those closest to us as well. Our past terror can cause us to lash out, be too attached, or not connected enough. The slew of issues that trauma can throw into our relationships with ourselves and others is endless. Therefore, we must understand our trauma's impact on our loved ones and everyone around us.

One way past trauma can affect our relationships is that it can lead us to become enmeshed with those we care about. We may not have healthy boundaries between us and the other person, and we can struggle to know who we are outside of the relationship. This can cause us to rely on others to make decisions for us, struggle to see that we have value on our own, and believe that we won't make it without someone else there at all times. This can make it hard for us to build up our self-esteem, and to be able to tap into how we are feeling. Relying completely on someone else can feel good at first, especially if we are exhausted by our PTSD and other life struggles, but enmeshed relationships are never good in the long run. They don't allow space for us to have our own experiences untainted by someone else, and they certainly don't help us rebuild our faith in ourselves and our ability to change and grow.

Trauma can also cause us to lash out at those around us in a rage because of all the pain we already feel inside. It's almost as if we just can't cope with the intensity of what we feel, and we snap at those we love or even get into fights when what we want is support. This tends to happen to those we are closest to because they are around us the most and checking in frequently. If we are caught off guard or on a bad day we can act out of our trauma experience, and yell, scream, blame, and shame. However, sometimes we do this to unsuspecting strangers, such as someone who cut us off on the highway, or a customer service representative on the phone. If we don't know how to healthily express the anger and upset we feel, it can erupt out of us at any time.

We can also use our relationships with others to initiate another traumatizing event. This can be through engaging in an abusive relationship just like the one we were in before, or by using the person to act out our terrorizing experiences as a way of taking the power back or being in control of it.

> My past trauma hasn't gotten in the way of any long-term relationships, but I did go through a period of time where I used sex with men as a form of punishment for myself and a way to cope with the trauma.

We can use our relationships to continue the pain or to create a new situation in which we are terrorized again, and I know that may sound odd; I mean, why would we want to harm ourselves again? However, there are many reasons we could do this; for example, we may not know what a healthy relationship looks like because no one in our life has shown us how to have one. We could think that the pain we feel is normal and a part of every relationship, or believe that we deserve to be in bad, hurtful relationships due to the shame caused by our trauma.

If our trauma occurred when we were young or happened as a result of a dysfunctional family (e.g., domestic violence or another form of abuse), we can grow up having skewed perceptions and beliefs about relationships. This can cause us to get into yet another abusive relationship because it's what feels comfortable and what has been modeled for us growing up. I know people often wonder why someone would stay in an abusive relationship, but if it's all that they know, and it's the way love and connection were shown to them as a child, it's natural that they would be drawn to it. They may find comfort in the abuse and the unpredictable behavior, because as we know, change can be uncomfortable and extremely difficult. On the flip side, being raised in an abusive home can lead to us being extremely cautious, jumping to conclusions when someone acts in a way that reminds us of our past. This can lead to us seeing other's actions in an unfavorable light, always assuming the worst. This overprotective state can cause us to act in emotionally abusive ways, making it difficult to have healthy and happy relationships, and possibly lead to being called toxic and hurtful.

Not to mention that being in a traumatic situation can also wear away at the relationship we have with ourselves. The shame,

And unfortunately, due to our upbringing, we didn't know what love looked like, or what healthy attachment was. I never had a parent I could go to, and neither did she. We became each other's everything. And with the shame involved, this was quite the recipe for disaster. And soon became a super abusive relationship. There were a lot of fistfights, and a lot of arguing, a lot of controlling each other, a lot of manipulation. It was pretty messy.

embarrassment, and guilt we can feel as a result of living through a traumatic experience can cause us to push everyone away to feel safe and ensure we don't upset anyone else. Since the world around us doesn't feel safe, we can shut it all out, giving ourselves complete control over our self-limited environment. I have had many patients take jobs where they can work from home, and disconnect from everyone else as a way of protecting themselves from another upset, sharing that they prefer to let their relationships go rather than work on them, because they can't stomach being to blame for anything else. While this makes sense when it comes to safety, it doesn't help us move past our trauma; it only broadens its reach, making everything dangerous. One of my patients told me that she built up these walls to keep herself safe, only to realize she had created her own prison. I thought that was a powerful visual to describe what this protective measure can do to us over time.

> I personally haven't been in any relationship during recovery, although I think it would help sometimes. It's tough being my own 'check in on her person.' It would be nice to simply have someone else around to say, 'Whoa, you are looking overwhelmed! Are you okay? Time to distract!' Or to simply help reground . . .

If we don't push everyone away and build up walls, we can believe we have to hide parts of ourselves from our friends and family so that they will accept us, sometimes even overcompensating by putting on a happy face and pretending everything is okay. I constantly hear how exhausting it can be to wear this happy mask all day at work, or that the pressure to be the "fun one" can be difficult when we were just triggered. Not being able to be ourselves or to let ourselves have down days can leave us feeling that no one knows who we are or what we are really going through, and that can be lonely and isolating too.

There are many ways that trauma can negatively affect our relationships, but I think that's enough of the doom and gloom. It's time to discuss the ways that we can get our relationships back on track, because with the right tools and techniques, they can improve and become the support we need on our path to recovery.

WAYS TO IMPROVE
OUR RELATIONSHIPS

Whether our relationships have been hindered by one or by all of the issues that can come along with a history of trauma, don't fret; with some simple strategies

> Even now that I've been diagnosed with PTSD, I haven't told my husband, or anyone really, because I feel the need to protect the people I love from having to deal with that, even though I know them being able to support me is what I need. I feel like I have to tackle it on my own and because of that have been slowly pushing people away, which has only been hurting my relationships with others, when in reality I'm trying to protect them for some reason.

and skills, we can get them to a healthy and helpful place. Doing this work is important because we need social support when healing from traumatic experiences, and even though we like to think we can go at it alone and just push through, having real loving support is vital to our recovery.

The first tip for improving our relationships is clear communication; and don't worry, everyone struggles at clearly communicating to others what's going on, how they are feeling, or what they need from other people. However, we can learn how to best do it and practice those skills until we feel more comfortable; trust me when I tell you that putting effort into doing this will improve all of your relationships, especially the one you have with yourself, so stick with it.

Before we get into sharing with others, we first have to figure out what it is we are feeling, thinking, and needing from them. I know we discussed this a bit before, but it's also important to mention it here, because we can't communicate about something we know nothing about. So, we need to get to know ourselves a bit: pay attention to our thoughts, beliefs, and what assistance could be helpful, and write that stuff down.

Once we have that information, we can decide what we need to share with our friends and family. My advice here is to keep it simple, focus on the issues that you know are affecting your relationship, and lean into the things you usually brush over—meaning that instead of acting as if things are okay, or bottling up how you feel only to explode later, let's talk about those patterns. Let them know that you have been traumatized, you are working on it in therapy, and you have become aware of the ways you may have taken it out on them. List some of the situations and things you did that you wish you didn't, and ask for forgiveness. Also, make sure you give space to their experience too; this isn't all about you and your struggles, it's about the relationship you have together. You need to make space for their upsets, too, and giving time for these types of real conversations will help you both heal and grow closer together. Not to mention that it can prevent you from bottling everything up, lying about how you are doing, or feeling pressure to put on a happy face when you aren't doing well. Being vulnerable in our relationships is the only way to feel truly supported and cared for; if we don't open up, those in our life won't know how to help. We need

> It was also difficult to learn to let people care about me and help me. Having supportive friends gives me people I can go to when I struggle and they can call me out when I am doing harm to myself. They understand trauma more now, so we can support each other on that level.

to give others a chance to listen and learn, and do our best to offer them the same in return.

Clear communication will also need to include conversations about our triggers and working to let others know what they are and when we have been upset by them. So often in relationships, we don't let someone know we are overwhelmed, but because this can cause us to lash out, freeze, or even have a panic attack, we need to let them know why it's happening and that it's not their fault. If we don't take the time to explain what's going on or let them learn along with us, they could think they're to blame, and get defensive or want to leave. We don't want a lack of vulnerability and understanding to cause more issues, and to prevent that from happening, we just have to try our best to let them know.

Another helpful tool in relationship building is healthy boundaries. We cannot make every conversation about us or always feel that we are giving to others without getting anything back. Healthy relationships operate with give and take. I know this can be difficult to calculate, and that's because we shouldn't be keeping a laundry list of all we have done versus what others have contributed. Instead, we should be taking the time to check in on ourselves and how we feel in certain relationships. Do we feel that the other person knows what's going on in our life? Do we know how they are doing and have listened to them share as well? After spending time with them, do we feel rejuvenated and good about things? Or not? All of these questions are important to check in on, and if something feels off, go back to the first tip and talk about it. Then, we can take some action to right the relationship so that it's healthy and beneficial to both parties. Even if the relationship is toxic, doing this exercise can help us more quickly recognize when things are off and feel more empowered to speak up about it.

When we have survived a traumatic experience, we can struggle to connect with ourselves and who we are, which can cause us to easily get sucked into relationships with people who will tell us what to think, do, and believe. This enmeshment can leave us without a sense of self, and while it may be comfortable for a while, we aren't able to process and move past our trauma in this state. Figuring out who we are, what we like, and what we don't like can take time and, just like recovery, it will be hard, but I cannot think of anything that will be more worth it. We need to do our best to consider what we want to do each day, what food sounds good, and who we want to spend our time with. Journaling is a great way to think through our options, consider situations where we wanted to speak up but didn't, and write out some ways we could be more assertive in the future. This introspection can allow us to sort through what is ours and what is someone else's, which can stop us from taking on someone else's pain and from blaming other people for how we feel. Setting up and maintaining boundaries can seem impossible at first, but just like any change, once we get over that initial disruption, we get comfortable in the new way of doing things, and before we know it, going back to an enmeshed situation will be difficult and unbearable.

>
> Learning to separate myself from my mother and see that it wasn't my fault helped a ton with my relationship to myself. Seeing I have value as a person.

Since trauma can cause us to think the world isn't safe and people aren't always good, intimacy of any kind can be tough to come by. It can be scary to let people in and allow them to get to know our true selves, which is why we often keep people at arm's length. However, to get the support we need, we are going to have to let people in, let them see us without our mask on, and share our real self. I know this isn't easy, but if we don't allow it, we will always feel alone and that no one understands what we are going through—because they don't. We cannot expect people to read our mind and know how to respond; we have to let them know what we are thinking and feeling and allow them to be there for us. Not everyone in our life deserves to know our most intimate details, but finding one person who cares for us, who we can trust, can be invaluable.

WHAT ABOUT SEXUAL INTIMACY?

Intimacy in relationships can be emotional and physical, and for those of us who have had sexual-based trauma, physical intimacy can feel impossible. Allowing someone to get that close, possibly doing similar things that our abuser did, can be triggering and unpleasant. This is why communication is imperative if we want to be able to engage in a healthy sexual relationship. I know talking about any past traumatic experience is uncomfortable, and talking about how it relates to our sex life, well, that could be excruciating, but it's the only way we can move past what happened and have healthy sexual experiences. Having a partner who will listen and work with us is going to be the most important part of this work.

The growth of our sexual relationships will take time, and they will need to be patient as we figure out our triggers, utilize grounding techniques so we don't constantly dissociate, and slowly prove to our brain and body that sex can be a loving and enjoyable act. While it's great to have a partner who is going to be there through this work, it's also important that we choose to do this because it's what we want, not just what our

I have been so thankful for my boyfriend who has been so supportive of me and my recovery. He's played a really important role and continues to by reminding me that I am safe now and I am enough. His support means the world to me. That being said it's also difficult focusing on trauma work and romantic relationships at once. Intimacy is a challenge for both of us in different ways that we continue to work on together.

partner wants. I only say this because I have had too many patients and viewers tell me that they wanted to work on their sexual intimacy because they were afraid their partner was going to leave if they didn't. I know this is hard to hear, but if someone is going to leave us because we aren't able to have a healthy sex life yet, let them go. This is going to be a painful process—starting and stopping sexual acts, struggling to feel safe, often dissociating—and we need someone there with us who wants to support us as we find our way. Anything less than that will only make this arduous process even more grueling.

By talking about what happened in therapy and with our partner, we can heal from our past sexual trauma and go on to have a healthy, happy sex life. One of my favorite tools to use to help move this along comes from *The Courage to Heal Workbook* and it has survivors put together safe sex guidelines, splitting up intimate acts into three categories: safe, possibly safe, and unsafe.[1] This can help guide us and our partner as we try other sexual acts together, starting with safe ones and moving on to possibly safe ones. This also gives us an entire section of things that aren't safe to share with our partner, so that they don't accidentally do something upsetting. I know a lot of this sounds slow and tedious, but to prove to ourselves that sex doesn't have to be about shame, control, or pain, we are going to have to take our time.

Another way to improve our sexual intimacy is to talk about it. I don't mean to talk about the trauma and our healing, but talk about sex with each other. We should feel open to share our fantasies, things we would like to try in the bedroom, or something our partner did that we liked. Sometimes we have to be more intentional about connecting with each other, and trying to start and engage in these conversations can not only allow us to learn more about our partner and what they like, but it also helps us to tap into our own sexual desires. I know this can be tough at first, but we should keep trying, maybe even journal about it a bit first so that we can find the right words for what we are thinking and feeling. And by continuing to go at our pace, talking about it along the way, and working with our sexual partner, we will be able to have a healthy and enjoyable sex life again.

HOW DO I FIND GOOD PEOPLE?

The most common issue my patients and viewers have with relationships is knowing who to have them with. As we discussed throughout this book, when we have been traumatized, it can be hard to know who to trust, and if we haven't had good experiences with people, we could have taken steps to isolate completely. However, having supportive loving relationships during our trauma recovery is incredibly important, and that's why I am going to share some of the ways we can figure out who we should build a relationship with.

The first step is to consider the traits that we enjoy in people. If that's too difficult, we can simply consider what characteristics our abusers or other toxic relationships had and write down the opposite. These can be things like being caring, supportive, trustworthy, calm, or even challenging. Once we have our list of possible qualities to look for, I would encourage you to bring it into your next therapy session and talk about it with your therapist. Whenever we are embarking on something that challenges an old way of thinking and acting, we want to check in with someone else to ensure we are doing it safely. If our therapist agrees that those traits are healthy and worthy of our time and energy, then we can reference this list as we meet new people, letting it be our new relationships guide.

The second step is to take our time getting to know people before we let them into our lives completely. This could mean that we only hang out with our coworkers in group settings so we are safe and have a chance to see how they interact with other people, or that we schedule weekly coffee dates to ensure it's during the day, and can be over once our coffee is gone. Any type of relationship will take time to build, and a healthy person isn't going to rush us into intimacy or dump a lot of personal information onto us right away. It's okay to not be available to hang out all the time, or taking a few hours to respond to a text. We want to build healthy boundaries from the beginning, and giving ourselves space to consider how our last get-together went is part of that. If we feel rushed or as if it's not okay to take our time, that's a red flag that this person doesn't respect us or our boundaries, and we should probably stop seeing them. Giving ourselves time to slowly get to know someone will leave space for these red flags to make themselves known. If we get too close too quickly, it can be even harder to end the relationship, so give ourselves time to slowly ease into it.

Finally, remember that we can end a relationship at any time. I know that sounds obvious, but too often we feel stuck in these toxic or abusive situations when all we have to do is stop responding to their calls and texts and end the relationship. I know surviving a traumatic experience can leave us feeling like something is wrong with us and we deserve bad things, but trust me when I tell you that we all deserve happy and healthy relationships. Since I know we can all talk ourselves in and out of relationships, and we often don't know what's healthy or not, here is a short and by no means an exhaustive list of reasons it's acceptable to end a relationship:

- They have hurt you emotionally, physically, or sexually, or have neglected you.
- They put you down, trash-talking you and those you love.
- They don't like you having other friends or spending time with your family.
- Spending time with them is exhausting and you dread it.
- They tell you what to do, how to spend your money, or who you can see.

- They are so easily upset; you find yourself walking on eggshells around them.
- They don't respect your boundaries and will ignore any assertion you make (e.g., you say you are not comfortable going somewhere and they expect you to go anyway).
- They only talk about themselves and never ask you how you are doing.
- They share your private information with other people without your permission.
- You don't want to be in a relationship with them anymore.

The only caveat to that short list is that if we are in a relationship with someone who is challenging us to speak up more and do our therapy homework, and they don't let us pretend everything is okay when it's not, well, that's not a reason to end it. We all need people in our life who know when we are lying and are there to support yet push us along in the right direction. I know it's uncomfortable, but all change feels that way, so check in with your therapist about it, and remember that relationships take some effort and a lot of vulnerability, but finding good people who know us well and can support us along the way is invaluable.

> Relational connection is key to feeling safe enough to remove the mask. It's key to feeling supported when you can't get your words out. It's key to reframing your thinking.
>
> It's key to finding hope when all seems lost.

KEY TAKEAWAYS

- Surviving a traumatic experience not only affects us but those around us.

- Our PTSD symptoms can damage our relationships. Some of the most common ways are lashing out in anger, isolating, struggling with boundaries and becoming enmeshed, using our relationships to continue the pain, skewing our perception of others, and allowing shame to ruin our faith in ourselves.

- We can fix our relationships through clear communication and healthy boundaries.

- Trauma can also make intimacy difficult, but by communicating with our partner, and being patient as we work through it, intimacy can get better.

- Creating a safe sex guideline of what is safe, possibly safe, and unsafe can prevent us from being retraumatized.

- To find people worth having in our lives we have to figure out what traits we desire in others, take our time getting to know them, and know that we can end a relationship at any time.

- Relationships are a key part of our recovery from trauma and will make the journey less painful and lonely.

EPILOGUE

I wish we lived in a world where bad things didn't happen and people were not traumatized by others, but unfortunately, that's not the case. Abuse, assault, school shootings, and much more are happening in our world each day, and surviving these traumatic experiences is no small feat. I want you to know that I see you, hear you, and know that this path to recovery can feel impossible at times. That's why I decided to write this book: to remind anyone out there who has been through a horrific experience that they are not alone and that with the right help, it can get better.

There is no judgment here, no expectations of when you should feel better or that you have to get into this difficult work right now. You are in control of your recovery and get to go at your own pace. I hope that you use this book in a way that suits you and your recovery process, and that it can be a reminder of the resources available when you are ready. Trauma already takes so much from us, but through the stories and therapeutic tools I hope you feel empowered to take back what is yours; placing boundaries where they need to be and putting yourself first.

Remember that you deserve to be free from PTSD symptoms and any feelings of shame. You are important, valued, and worthy of love. Keep putting one foot in front of the other, pushing back against the lies you were told in the past. You can live a life free from the concern of what happened and instead have focus and excitement for what tomorrow can bring. Trust me, I have seen it happen over and over again, and it can happen for you too.

NOTES

CHAPTER 1: OUR SHARED TRAUMA:
HOW SOCIAL MEDIA AFFECTS OUR MENTAL HEALTH

1. Pew Research Center, "About Three-in-Ten U.S. Adults Say They Are 'Almost Constantly' Online," July 2019, https://www.pew research.org/fact-tank/2019/07/25/americans-going-online -almost-constantly/.
2. D. J. Kuss and M. D. Griffiths, "Social Networking Sites and Addiction: Ten Lessons Learned," *International Journal of Environmental Research and Public Health* 14, no. 3 (2017): 311, https://doi.org/10.3390/ijerph14030311.
3. P. Fossion et al., "Family Approach with Grandchildren of Holocaust Survivors," *American Journal of Psychotherapy* 57, no. 4 (2003): 519–527.

CHAPTER 2: HAVE I BEEN TRAUMATIZED?
PTSD & WHAT YOU NEED TO KNOW

1. G. C. Bunn, A. D. Lovie, and G. D. Richards, eds., *Psychology in Britain: Historical Essays and Personal Reflections* (Leicester, UK: BPS Books, 2001).
2. Edgar Jones, "Shell Shocked," *American Psychological Association* 43, no. 6 (June 2012), https://www.apa.org/monitor/2012/06 /shell-shocked.
3. Jones, "Shell Shocked."
4. Jones, "Shell Shocked."

5. Bessel van der Kolk, *The Body Keeps the Score: Brain, Mind, and Body in the Healing of Trauma* (New York: Viking, 2014).
6. American Psychiatric Association, *Diagnostic and Statistical Manual of Mental Disorders*, 5th ed. (Washington, DC: American Psychiatric Association Publishing, 2013).
7. *Diagnostic and Statistical Manual of Mental Disorders*.
8. *Diagnostic and Statistical Manual of Mental Disorders*.

CHAPTER 3: WHAT CAN CAUSE PTSD?

1. American Psychiatric Association, *Diagnostic and Statistical Manual of Mental Disorders*, 5th ed. (Washington, DC: American Psychiatric Association Publishing, 2013).
2. *Diagnostic and Statistical Manual of Mental Disorders*.

CHAPTER 4: WHAT IS DISSOCIATION & WHY DOES IT HAPPEN?

1. American Psychiatric Association, *Diagnostic and Statistical Manual of Mental Disorders*, 5th ed. (Washington, DC: American Psychiatric Association Publishing, 2013).
2. *Diagnostic and Statistical Manual of Mental Disorders*, 292.
3. S. Sexton and R. Natale, "Risks and Benefits of Pacifiers," *American Family Physician* 79, no. 8 (2009): 681–685.

CHAPTER 5: WHAT IS REPEATED TRAUMA? C-PTSD & HOW IT'S DIFFERENT

1. Patrick J. Carnes and Bonnie Phillips, *The Betrayal Bond: Breaking Free of Exploitative Relationships*, rev. ed. (Boca Raton, FL: HCI, 2019).
2. Nielsen, "Rebalancing the 'COVID-19 Effect' on Alcohol Sales," 2020, https://www.nielsen.com/us/en/insights/article/2020/rebalancing-the-covid-19-effect-on-alcohol-sales/.

CHAPTER 6: ARE WE SURE IT'S C-PTSD?

1. American Psychiatric Association, *Diagnostic and Statistical Manual of Mental Disorders*, 5th ed. (Washington, DC: American Psychiatric Association Publishing, 2013).
2. *Diagnostic and Statistical Manual of Mental Disorders*.
3. *Diagnostic and Statistical Manual of Mental Disorders*.
4. *Diagnostic and Statistical Manual of Mental Disorders*.
5. *Diagnostic and Statistical Manual of Mental Disorders*.
6. *Diagnostic and Statistical Manual of Mental Disorders*.
7. *Diagnostic and Statistical Manual of Mental Disorders*.
8. *Diagnostic and Statistical Manual of Mental Disorders*.
9. *Diagnostic and Statistical Manual of Mental Disorders*.
10. *Diagnostic and Statistical Manual of Mental Disorders*.
11. M. S. Harned, "The Combined Treatment of PTSD with Borderline Personality Disorder," *Current Treatment Options in Psychiatry* 1 (2014): 335–344, https://doi.org/10.1007/s40501-014-0025-2.
12. Marylène Cloitre et al., "Distinguishing PTSD, Complex PTSD, and Borderline Personality Disorder: A Latent Class Analysis," *European Journal of Psychotraumatology* 5, no. 1 (2014): 25097, https://doi.org/10.3402/ ejpt.v5.25097.
13. Gordon H. Bower, ed., *The Psychology of Learning and Motivation: Advances in Research and Theory* (Academic Press, 1981), 30.

CHAPTER 7: WHAT ARE THE 4 ATTACHMENT STYLES? WHY TRAUMA IS ROOTED IN CHILDHOOD

1. Substance Abuse and Mental Health Services Administration, "Understanding Child Trauma," April 29, 2020, https://www.samhsa.gov/child-trauma/understanding-child-trauma.
2. V. J. Felitti et al., "Relationship of Childhood Abuse and Household Dysfunction to Many of the Leading Causes of Death in

Adults: The Adverse Childhood Experiences (ACE) Study," *American Journal of Preventive Medicine* 14, no. 4 (1998): 245–258, https://doi.org/10.1016/S0749-3797(98)00017-8.

3. Felitti et al., "Relationship of Childhood Abuse and Household Dysfunction."

4. Joining Forces for Children, "What Are ACEs?" 2020, http://www.joiningforcesforchildren.org/what-are-aces/.

5. Nadine Burke Harris, "How Childhood Trauma Affects Health Across a Lifetime," TED Talks, September 2014, https://www.ted.com/talks/nadine_burke_harris_how_childhood_trauma_affects_health_across_a_lifetime?language=en#t-362018.

6. S. W. Porges, "The Polyvagal Theory: New Insights into Adaptive Reactions of the Autonomic Nervous System," *Cleveland Clinic Journal of Medicine* 76, suppl. 2 (2009): S86–S90, https://doi.org/10.3949/ccjm.76.s2.17.

7. John Bowlby, *Attachment and Loss* (New York: Basic Books, 1969).

8. S. A. McLeod, "Mary Ainsworth," Simply Psychology, August 5, 2018, https://www.simplypsychology.org/mary-ainsworth.html.

9. M. D. S. Ainsworth et al., *Patterns of Attachment: A Psychological Study of the Strange Situation* (Hillsdale, NJ: Erlbaum, 1978).

10. M. Main and J. Solomon, "Procedures for Identifying Infants as Disorganized/Disoriented During the Ainsworth Strange Situation," in *Attachment in the Preschool Years: Theory, Research, and Intervention*, ed. M. T. Greenberg, D. Cicchetti, and E. M. Cummings (Chicago: University of Chicago Press, 1990), 121–160.

11. Marsha Linehan, *DBT Skills Training Handouts and Worksheets* (New York: Guilford Press, 2015).

12. Linehan, *DBT Skills Training Handouts and Worksheets*.

13. Linehan, *DBT Skills Training Handouts and Worksheets*.

CHAPTER 8: CAN TRAUMA BE PASSED DOWN?
TRANSGENERATIONAL TRAUMA AND ITS LASTING EFFECTS

1. M. Heurich et al., "Country, Cover or Protection: What Shapes the Distribution of Red Deer and Roe Deer in the Bohemian Forest Ecosystem?" *PLoS ONE* 10, no. 3 (2015): e0120960, https://doi.org/10.1371/journal.pone.0120960.

2. P. Fossion et al., "Family Approach with Grandchildren of Holocaust Survivors," *American Journal of Psychotherapy* 57, no. 4 (2003): 519–527.

3. B. Bezo and S. Maggi, "Intergenerational Perceptions of Mass Trauma's Impact on Physical Health and Well-Being," *Psychological Trauma: Theory, Research, Practice, and Policy* 10, no. 1 (January 2018).

4. B. Dias and K. Ressler, "Parental Olfactory Experience Influences Behavior and Neural Structure in Subsequent Generations," *Nature Neuroscience* 17 (2014): 89–96, https://doi.org/10.1038/nn.3594.

5. N. A. Youssef et al., "The Effects of Trauma, with or without PTSD, on the Transgenerational DNA Methylation Alterations in Human Offsprings," *Brain Sciences* 8, no. 5 (2018): 83, https://doi.org/10.3390/brainsci8050083.

6. F. A. Champagne, "Epigenetic Mechanisms and the Transgenerational Effects of Maternal Care," *Frontiers in Neuroendocrinology* 29, no. 3 (2008): 386–397, https://doi.org/10.1016/j.yfrne.2008.03.003.

7. Centers for Disease Control and Prevention, "Corona Disease 2019 (COVID-19): Cases in the U.S. June 24th, 2020," https://www.cdc.gov/coronavirus/2019-ncov/cases-updates/cases-in-us.html.

8. J. P. Daniels, "Colombian Designers Prepare Cardboard Hospital Beds That Double as Coffins," *Guardian*, May 27, 2020, https://www.theguardian.com/world/2020/may/27/colombia-coronavirus-cardboard-hospital-beds-coffins.

9. S. W. Porges, "The Polyvagal Theory: New Insights into Adaptive Reactions of the Autonomic Nervous System," *Cleveland Clinic Journal of Medicine* 76, suppl. 2 (2009): S86–S90, https://doi .org/10.3949/ccjm.76.s2.17.

10. P. A. Levine, *In an Unspoken Voice: How The Body Releases Trauma and Restores Goodness* (Berkeley, CA: North Atlantic Books, 2010).

CHAPTER 9: WHY DO WE FEEL SO SCARED?
THE SCIENCE OF TRAUMA MEMORIES

1. Michael Yassa, "Hippocampus," Encyclopædia Britannica, November 28, 2018, https://www.britannica.com/science /hippocampus.

2. University of Queensland Brain Institute, "How Are Memories Formed?" July 23, 2018, https://qbi.uq.edu.au/brain-basics/memory /how-are-memories-formed.

3. Bessel van der Kolk, *The Body Keeps the Score: Brain, Mind, and Body in the Healing of Trauma* (New York: Viking, 2014), 178.

4. Matthew P. Walker, "The Role of Slow Wave Sleep in Memory Processing," *Journal of Clinical Sleep Medicine* 5, no. 2 suppl. (2009): S20–S26.

5. Matthew Walker, "The Joe Rogan Experience. Joe Rogan Experience #1109—Matthew Walker," April 25, 2018, https://youtube .com/watch?v=/pwaWilO_Pig.

6. E. Joseph LeDoux, "Coming to Terms with Fear," *Proceedings of the National Academy of Sciences* 111, no. 8 (February 2014): 2871–2878, https://doi.org/10.1073/pnas.1400335111.

7. L. Cahill and J. L. McGaugh, "Mechanisms of Emotional Arousal and Lasting Declarative Memory," *Trends in Neurosciences* 21, no. 7 (1998): 294–299.

8. van der Kolk, *The Body Keeps the Score*, 178.

9. American Psychiatric Association, *Diagnostic and Statistical Manual of Mental Disorders*, 5th ed. (Washington, DC: American Psychiatric Association Publishing, 2013), 271.

10. Ashley Pettus, "Repressed Memory," *Harvard Magazine*, January–February 2008, https://www.harvardmagazine.com/2008/01/repressed-memory.html.

CHAPTER 10: HOW CAN WE RECOVER?
THE BENEFITS OF NEUROPLASTICITY

1. G. Berlucchi, "The Origin of the Term Plasticity in the Neurosciences: Ernesto Lugaro and Chemical Synaptic Transmission," *Journal of the History of the Neurosciences* 11, no. 3 (2002): 305–309, https://doi.org/10.1076/jhin.11.3.305.10396.

2. Saul McLeod, "Pavlov's Dogs," Simply Psychology, 2018, https://www.simplypsychology.org/pavlov.html.

3. Saul McLeod, "Skinner—Operant Conditioning," Simply Psychology, 2018, https://www.simplypsychology.org/operant-conditioning.html.

4. David D. Burns, *The Feeling Good Handbook* (New York: Plume, 1999).

CHAPTER 11: THE FOUNDATION OF HEALING:
FINDING THE RIGHT TREATMENT

1. M. L. Van Etten and S. Taylor, "Comparative Efficacy of Treatments for Post-Traumatic Stress Disorder: A Meta-Analysis," *Clinical Psychology & Psychotherapy* 5, no. 3 (1998).

2. "Trauma-Focused Cognitive Behavioral Therapy for Children Affected by Sexual Abuse or Trauma," Child Welfare Information Gateway, 2012, 6, https://www.childwelfare.gov/pubPDFs/trauma.pdf.

3. J. Kaplan and D. Tolin, "Exposure Therapy for Anxiety Disorders," *Psychiatric Times*, September 6, 2011, https://www.psychiatrictimes.com/view/exposure-therapy-anxiety-disorders.

4. Cognitive Behavior Therapy Center, "Schemas in Schema Therapy," 2020, http://cognitivebehaviortherapycenter.com/schema-therapy-california/schemas-in-schema-therapy/.

5. Eugene Lipov, "Using Stellate Ganglion Block (SGB) to Treat Post-Traumatic Stress Disorder," February 8, 2019, https://www.anxiety.org/stellate-ganglion-block-sgb-for-ptsd-research-update.

6. Christa McIntyre, "Is There a Role for Vagus Nerve Stimulation in the Treatment of Posttraumatic Stress Disorder?" *Bioelectronic in Medicine* 1, no. 2 (May 25, 2018), https://doi.org/10.2217/bem-2018-0002.

7. Butler Hospital, "How Does TMS Work?" 2020, http://www.butler.org/programs/outpatient/how-does-tms-work.cfm#:~:text=TMS%20uses%20a%20small%20electromagnetic,resonance%20imaging%20(MRI)%20machine.

CHAPTER 13: BREAKING THE CYCLE:
AVOIDING FUTURE TRAUMA & TRIGGERS

1. B. Sissons, "Exposure Therapy: What It Is and What to Expect," *Medical News Today*, May 5, 2020, https://www.medicalnewstoday.com/articles/exposure-therapy.

2. V. J. Harber and J. R. Sutton, "Endorphins and Exercise," *Sports Medicine* 1 (1984): 154–171, https://doi.org/10.2165/00007256-1984 01020-00004.

3. Adapted from "How to Use the Impulse Control Log" by S.A.F.E. Alternatives (2007–2020), https://selfinjury.com/resources/how-to-use-the-impulse-control-log/.

CHAPTER 14: RESILIENCE: BUILDING IT & KEEPING IT

1. Marsha Linehan, *DBT Skills Training Handouts and Worksheets* (New York: Guilford Press, 2015).

CHAPTER 15 : BUILDING SUPPORT:
HOW TO HAVE HEALTHY RELATIONSHIPS

1. Laura Davis, *The Courage to Heal Workbook: For Women and Men Survivors of Child Sexual Abuse* (New York: Harper, 1990).